CANCER ETIOLOGY, DIAGNOSIS AND TREATMENTS

DIETARY FLAVONOIDS INTERFERE WITH CANCER RADIOTHERAPY

CANCER ETIOLOGY, DIAGNOSIS AND TREATMENTS

Additional books and e-books in this series can be found on Nova's website under the Series tab.

CANCER ETIOLOGY, DIAGNOSIS AND TREATMENTS

DIETARY FLAVONOIDS INTERFERE WITH CANCER RADIOTHERAPY

KATRIN SAK

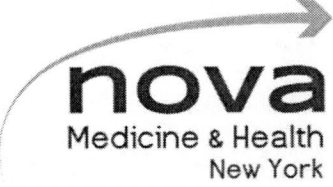

Copyright © 2019 by Nova Science Publishers, Inc.

All rights reserved. No part of this book may be reproduced, stored in a retrieval system or transmitted in any form or by any means: electronic, electrostatic, magnetic, tape, mechanical photocopying, recording or otherwise without the written permission of the Publisher.

We have partnered with Copyright Clearance Center to make it easy for you to obtain permissions to reuse content from this publication. Simply navigate to this publication's page on Nova's website and locate the "Get Permission" button below the title description. This button is linked directly to the title's permission page on copyright.com. Alternatively, you can visit copyright.com and search by title, ISBN, or ISSN.

For further questions about using the service on copyright.com, please contact:
Copyright Clearance Center
Phone: +1-(978) 750-8400   Fax: +1-(978) 750-4470   E-mail: info@copyright.com.

NOTICE TO THE READER

The Publisher has taken reasonable care in the preparation of this book, but makes no expressed or implied warranty of any kind and assumes no responsibility for any errors or omissions. No liability is assumed for incidental or consequential damages in connection with or arising out of information contained in this book. The Publisher shall not be liable for any special, consequential, or exemplary damages resulting, in whole or in part, from the readers' use of, or reliance upon, this material. Any parts of this book based on government reports are so indicated and copyright is claimed for those parts to the extent applicable to compilations of such works.

Independent verification should be sought for any data, advice or recommendations contained in this book. In addition, no responsibility is assumed by the Publisher for any injury and/or damage to persons or property arising from any methods, products, instructions, ideas or otherwise contained in this publication.

This publication is designed to provide accurate and authoritative information with regard to the subject matter covered herein. It is sold with the clear understanding that the Publisher is not engaged in rendering legal or any other professional services. If legal or any other expert assistance is required, the services of a competent person should be sought. FROM A DECLARATION OF PARTICIPANTS JOINTLY ADOPTED BY A COMMITTEE OF THE AMERICAN BAR ASSOCIATION AND A COMMITTEE OF PUBLISHERS.

Additional color graphics may be available in the e-book version of this book.

Library of Congress Cataloging-in-Publication Data

ISBN: 978-1-53616-708-1
Library of Congress Control Number:2019953058

Published by Nova Science Publishers, Inc. † New York

CONTENTS

Preface		vii
Introduction		ix
Abbreviations		xiii
Chapter 1	The Role of Radiotherapy in Cancer Treatment: Current Opportunities and Challenges	1
Chapter 2	Radiotherapy-Induced Cellular Responses: Major Mechanisms Behind Radioresistance	5
Chapter 3	Plant Flavonoids as Potential Dietary Radiosensitizers	17
Chapter 4	Modulation of Radiotherapeutic Efficacy by Dietary Flavonoids	21
Chapter 5	Conclusion and Further Challenges	105
References		109
About the Author		121
Index		123
Related Nova Publications		129

PREFACE

In parallel with the continuous rise of cancer incidence, the efficient treatment becomes an increasingly important public health concern. Radiotherapy has remained one of the most important anticancer approaches for clinical management of a variety of human tumors, as at least half of all oncological patients receive this therapy at some stages of their disease. With the hope to attain greater anticancer response, the interest in using natural plant-derived products as complementary treatments to conventional radiotherapy is substantially increased in the recent years. However, the interactions between phytochemicals and ionizing radiation are not always known and can be often unpredictable. Therefore, in this book, the current findings about the combined treatments of malignant cells with radiation and flavonoids, the largest group of human dietary plant polyphenols, are described. These data show that under carefully chosen dosage-schedule regimens, certain flavonoids or their natural mixtures can behave as potent radiosensitizers, augmenting radiotherapeutic efficacy in different preclinical cancer models. Such radiosensitizing action of flavonoids can be achieved through modulation of the redox status and suppression of several cellular survival pathways activated by radiotherapy, ultimately leading to the death of malignant cells. As flavonoids can concurrently protect normal healthy cells from irradiation-induced injury and thereby minimize toxic adverse reactions, use of these plant-derived agents as complementary approach to radiotherapy might open new avenues for enhancement of clinical outcome. Therefore, combining conventional anticancer modalities with conscious intake of flavonoid supplements as adjuvant agents might be an important future strategy to boost the therapeutic success in the treatment of various human malignancies.

INTRODUCTION

Cancer is a growing health problem and the second leading cause of death for both men and women all over the world, just after cardiovascular diseases. There were an estimated 18.1 million new cancer cases and 9.6 million cancer deaths in 2018 worldwide [1]. If the current industrial growth, environmental pollution and prevalence of unhealthy lifestyles will not slow down, the number of new cancer cases is expected to increase to 24.1 million annually by 2030 and to 29.5 million by 2040 [2]. Additionally, the aging of population also confers the rise in the number of patients with clinically significant malignant neoplasms.

As incidence of malignant disorders continuously increases, the development of their effective treatment becomes more and more important. Being a multifactorial disease, cancer requires also multimodal therapy, with radiotherapy as one of the major methods used to treat various human malignancies, either alone or in combination with other anticancer modalities, i.e., surgical resection and chemotherapy. In fact, more than 50% of newly diagnosed cancer patients receive radiation treatment at some stage of their disease [3]. However, the clinical concern of this therapeutic approach involves intrinsic or acquired radioresistance, as the success of radiotherapy is largely dependent on the radiosensitivity of tumoral cells. Therefore, overcoming radioresistance is a central issue for efficient application of radiotherapy.

To enhance the efficacy of conventional radiotherapy, the development of agents that sensitize cancerous cells to ionizing radiation or so-called radiosensitizers is a crucial task. There are two main requirements for such substances: first, they must selectively potentiate the radiation-induced killing of malignant cells to ultimately overcome radioresistance and improve therapeutic outcome; and secondly, these agents should not cause any harm to surrounding normal tissues and preferably protect them from radiation-induced injury [4, 5]. A number of recent studies have suggested that some dietary phytochemicals, such as curcumin derived from turmeric, resveratrol from grapes and gossypol isolated from cottonseed, can affect the radiotherapeutic efficacy, leading to enhanced responsiveness of tumor cells to ionizing radiation through targeting various cellular mechanisms [6]. However, although combination of radiotherapy with certain plant-derived polyphenols might become an important novel strategy to improve the therapeutic outcome in the future clinical settings, using diverse natural products as nutritional supplements by cancer patients undergoing radiotherapy has been an intriguing and provocative issue for years. Consumption of complementary treatments, including over-the-counter nutritional supplements and herbs, is rather prevalent among oncological patients in the course of their conventional anticancer therapies [7, 8], posing a question about the safety and actual interactions of the bioactive constituents with irradiation.

To through some light on this exciting topic, current findings about the combinatorial effects of radiation and flavonoids, the largest class of dietary plant polyphenols, are compiled in this book. These plant secondary metabolites are especially attractive considering their safety profile, proven through exposure of mankind to plant food items rich in flavonoids already for millennia. As flavonoids can target multiple key molecules and affect cellular survival signaling pathways [9, 10], these dietary agents could potentially act as novel candidates to regulate radiation-induced events and potentiate anticancer response when administered along with irradiation. Numerous preclinical findings presented in this book indeed suggest that flavonoids could be developed as potent radiosensitizers to improve the therapeutic efficacy and enhance clinical outcome of patients suffering from different tumors. Thereat, the structures of flavonoid lead compounds might provide the basis for further design of novel more efficient and specific semisynthetic inhibitors for combating radioresistance phenotype of human malignancies. As interactions between dietary flavonoids and radiotherapy represent a rather new research topic, the number of original studies is still relatively low today. However, considering the popularity and high interest in this subject, a large increase in publications could be expected in the near future. It is hoped that these new investigations will give further promise to cancer patients in developing more efficient and successful combinatorial strategies using flavonoids as adjuvant treatments for radiotherapy, with lower adverse reactions, prolonged survival time and improved quality of life.

ABBREVIATIONS

Akt	protein kinase B
APE1/Ref-1	apurinic/apyrimidinic endonuclease 1/redox factor-1
AR	androgen receptor
ARE	antioxidant response element
ATM	ataxia telangiectasia mutated
Bax	Bcl-2-associated X protein
Bcl-2	B-cell lymphoma 2
Bcl-xL	B-cell lymphoma-extra large
bw	body weight
CAT	catalase
CCK-8	Cell Counting Kit-8
Cdc2	cell division control protein 2
Chk2	checkpoint kinase 2
CHOP	CCAAT/enhancer binding protein homologous protein
COX-2	cyclooxygenase-2
CSC	cancer stem cell
cyt c	cytochrome c
DNA-PK	DNA-dependent protein kinase
DR	death receptor

Abbreviations

DSB	double-strand break
EGCG	epigallocatechin 3-gallate
EGFR	epidermal growth factor receptor
EMT	epithelial-mesenchymal transition
eNOS	endothelial NOS
ER	estrogen receptor
ERK	extracellular signal-regulated kinase
ERα	estrogen receptor-α
ERβ	estrogen receptor-β
GLUT-1	glucose transporter-1
GPx	glutathione peroxidase
GSH	glutathione
GST	glutathione S-transferase
Gy	gray
h	hour
HGF	hepatocyte growth factor
HIF-1α	hypoxia inducible factor-1α
HO1	heme oxygenase-1
HPV	human papillomavirus
HRR	homologous recombination
HRS	hyper-radiosensitivity
i.m.	intramuscular
i.p.	intraperitoneal
i.v.	intravenous
IAP	inhibitor of apoptosis protein
IGF1R	insulin-like growth factor 1 receptor
IL-6	interleukin-6
iNOS	inducible form of NOS
Keap1	Kelch-like ECH-associated protein 1
KRAS	Kirsten rat sarcoma viral oncogene
MAPK	mitogen-activated protein kinase
Mcl-1	myeloid cell leukemia-1
min	minutes
miR	microRNA

MMP	matrix metalloproteinase
MnSOD	manganese superoxide dismutase
MTS	3-(4,5-dimethylthiazol-2-yl)-5-(3-carboxymethoxyphenyl)-2-(4-sulfophenyl)-2H-tetrazolium
MTT	3-(4,5-dimethylthiazol-2-yl)-2,5-diphenyltetrazolium bromide
NF-κB	nuclear factor-κB
NHEJ	non-homologous end joining
nM	nanomolar
NO	nitric oxide
NOS	nitric oxide synthase
Nox2	NADPH oxidase 2
NQO1	NAD(P)H quinone oxidoreductase-1
Nrf2	nuclear factor erythroid 2-related factor 2
pAkt	phosphorylated Akt
PARP	poly (ADP-ribose) polymerase
PCNA	proliferating cell nuclear antigen
PGE2	prostaglandin E2
PI3K	phosphatidylinositol 3-kinase
PKB	protein kinase B
pRb	retinoblastoma protein
PTEN	phosphatase and tensin homolog
ROS	reactive oxygen species
RTK	receptor tyrosine kinase
s.c.	subcutaneous
SOD	superoxide dismutase
SRB	sulforhodamine B
STAT3	signal transducer and activator of transcription 3
TBARS	thiobarbituric acid reactive substances
TK1	thymidine kinase 1
TNF-α	tumor necrosis factor-α
uPA	urokinase-type plasminogen activator
VEGF	vascular endothelial growth factor

wt	wild type
XIAP	X-linked inhibitor of apoptosis protein
μM	micromolar

Chapter 1

THE ROLE OF RADIOTHERAPY IN CANCER TREATMENT: CURRENT OPPORTUNITIES AND CHALLENGES

Cancer is the second leading cause of global death, just behind cardiovascular disorders, whereas its incidence rate is continuously rising each year [11, 12]. The major risk factors of this multifactorial disease are related to the environment and lifestyle of individuals [6, 13]. Cancer is a multistage process revealing numerous defects in molecular mechanisms responsible for cell growth, survival and death [6]. Cancer therapy has remained as complex as the disease itself, consisting mainly of surgery, chemotherapy and radiotherapy; being exploited in accordance with the type, location, size and stage of the tumor, but considering also the age and general medical condition of the patient [6, 12, 14]. Ionizing radiation therapy as one of the mainstream anticancer modalities in the current clinical settings has been used to manage malignancies already for more than hundred years [6]. At least half of cancer patients use this therapeutic option at some stage of their disease [3, 6, 11, 15].

Radiotherapy is currently applied for the treatment of localized tumors of various types of malignancies, including brain, lung, prostatic, breast, cervical and pancreatic cancers, but also leukemias and lymphomas [6, 16-18]. Compared to the systemic effects of chemotherapy to a wide range of tissues, radiotherapy represents a more localized treatment approach, thereby preserving normal healthy tissues [6, 12, 19]. However, although localized prostate cancer is sensitive to conventional radiotherapy, this treatment is insufficient to eradicate all tumoral cells in a significant proportion of patients and residual disease often causes clinical relapse and disease progression [20-23]. Moreover, prostate irradiation affects also the adjacent normal structures, especially bladder neck, penile bulk, and the anterior rectal wall, resulting in adverse reactions in urinary, erectile and intestinal functions and lowering quality of life of men [24]. Thoracic radiotherapy plays a critical role in the management of patients with early-stage and locally advanced inoperable non-small cell lung cancers, but therapeutic outcomes are often unsatisfactory, local tumor control is poor and risk for recurrences is high [25-29]. In addition, radiation-induced interstitial pulmonary inflammation (pneumonitis) and fibrosis can be accompanied by thoracic radiotherapy even in up to 30% of patients, affecting breathing and reducing quality of life [29, 30]. Radiotherapy remains a mainstream treatment strategy also for patients with unresectable and locally advanced esophageal squamous cell carcinoma [31, 32], gastric cancer [33] and oral squamous cell carcinoma [34]. For early stage cervical cancer, the disease can be treated with radiation or surgery with almost equivalent results [35]. Irradiation plays an important role also as adjuvant therapy in reducing the disease recurrence and improving disease-free and overall survival rates after surgical resection (and/or chemotherapy) for patients with different solid tumors, such as cervical cancer [36], breast cancer [17], colorectal cancer [37, 38], bladder cancer [39] or malignant brain tumors [40, 41]. Unfortunately, 90% of glioblastoma patients receiving radiotherapy after tumor resection still develop recurrence in the proximity of the primary neoplastic site, making gliomas most insusceptible neoplasms to irradiation regimens [40, 42].

Therefore, although radiotherapy is one of the most effective modalities in the management of malignant disorders, its application is often restricted by two major concerns. First, successful treatment of cancer by radiotherapy depends to a great extent on the sensitivity of malignant cells to ionizing radiation. However, a large number of tumor cells respond only poorly (or do not respond) to irradiation or lose their susceptibility in the course of treatment [12, 43, 44]. Such intrinsic or acquired radioresistance is considered as one of the major reasons for therapeutic failure, local recurrence, progression and distant metastasis [12, 19]. Indeed, glioblastoma and pancreatic cancer are considered as intrinsically radioresistant malignancies; whereas for most tumor types, resistance becomes more serious when tumors relapse, regardless of their original radioresponsiveness [15]. Moreover, treatment-induced resistance to radiation is characterized by enhanced invasive and metastatic character of surviving radioresistant tumor cells, which makes their clinical management even more difficult and forces the physician to either increase the radiation doses or change the treatment modality [6, 33, 42, 45]. Second, ionizing radiation does not affect only target malignant cells but induces dose-related toxicity also in the surrounding normal tissues leading to severe adverse side effects and thereby limiting therapeutic outcome [12, 43, 46, 47]. Thus, selective killing of malignant cells without harming nearby normal cells is the principle challenge in radiotherapy.

Accordingly, identification and development of agents that sensitize tumor tissues to radiation or so-called radiosensitizers are required to improve radiotherapeutic efficacy, i.e., to reduce the radioresistance influence and augment the degree of tumor damage by minimizing radiation dose and sparing neighboring normal tissues [4, 6, 12, 28, 47]. One approach for this is to combine radiotherapy with traditional anticancer drugs that affect tumor characteristics and microenvironment, such as 5-fluorouracil, taxanes and non-steroidal antiinflammatory agents. As these treatment modalities act via different mechanisms, it is expected that their combination might enhance radioresponsiveness of cancer cells and strengthen therapeutic outcomes. However, the specificity toward malignant cells has remained poor and injury of normal cells is increased by addition of cytotoxic chemotherapeutics [4, 6, 27, 28, 48-50]. Therefore, development of novel more effective and less toxic radiosensitizers remains a high priority and is of clinical importance, still demanding lots of efforts. Naturally occurring agents that are non-toxic and safe to the human beings are certainly preferred in the searching process of effective radiosensitizers.

Chapter 2

RADIOTHERAPY-INDUCED CELLULAR RESPONSES: MAJOR MECHANISMS BEHIND RADIORESISTANCE

Radiotherapy delivers high energy radiation, primarily X-rays, to predefined tumor mass with the aim to kill cancer cells [6, 31]. Radiation is usually given in several fractions rather than as a single dose to allow normal cells the space of time to recover between each therapy session, thereby minimizing the damage to normal tissues and undesirable side effects [6]. The damage caused by ionizing radiation to the exposed cells is either direct by interacting with macromolecules, such as DNA, and causing DNA strand breaks, or indirect by colliding with water molecules and leading to generation of free radical species, such as reactive oxygen species (ROS) inside the tumor cells [6, 8, 51] (Figure 1). Irradiation is known to initiate various signaling pathways involved in processes governing both cell survival and cell death, including DNA repair, cell cycle transition, changes in redox signaling, survival mechanisms and apoptotic pathways. Balance between these events and alterations in the activity of respective cascades are responsible for the ultimate effect of radiotherapy in the cells [6, 48, 52, 53]. Moreover, the development of unresponsiveness to ionizing radiation is also determined by these cellular mediators, whereas affecting the target molecules would be an effective way to combat the problems of radioresistance. As signaling pathways which promote cellular survival could result in radioresistance, their inhibition before irradiation is expected to gain the full therapeutic benefit [16]. However, the exact molecular mechanisms and cellular factors behind the radioresistance phenomenon are not completely clear [28, 42, 54, 55]. Improvement of the antitumor effects and therapeutic outcome of radiotherapy is of high clinical significance; hence, elucidation of these mechanisms, identification of molecular biomarkers and possibilities to interfere with radiosensitizers have remained crucial fields of research [4, 27, 56, 57].

The most frequently used biological systems in the experimental cancer studies involve cell lines isolated from malignant tissues. Although *in vitro* radiosensitizing potency of testing agents is traditionally assessed by clonogenic capacity, cellular proliferation studies are also important. Application of clonogenic assay is not feasible in cell lines with no or only minimal colony-forming capacity and in primary cells derived from tumor biopsies; in suspension-growing lines its execution is technically very complicated. Moreover, whereas clonogenic capacity characterizes the self-renewal potency and regrowth of single tumor cells revealing thereby the *in vivo* chance of tumor recurrence, proliferation represents rather the bulk of the overall malignant cell population. Both aspects have valuable implications for cancer therapy and are therefore used in the experiments studying potential novel radiosensitizers [58].

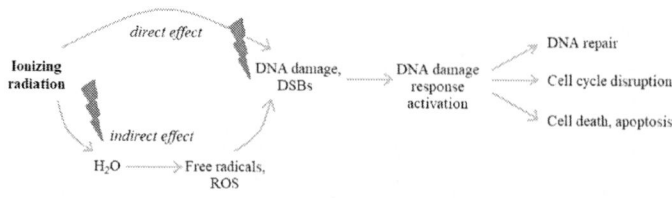

Figure 1. Major mechanisms followed by ionizing radiation of cancer cells.

2.1. REDOX SIGNALING

Generation of ROS and oxidative stress is one of the major killing mechanisms of ionizing radiation therapy [31, 39, 44, 59, 60]. Although ROS are usually regarded as host defensive molecules against different exogenous pathogens, excessive ROS produced by water ionization within radiolysis cause breakdown of double-stranded DNA and damage cellular proteins and biomembranes, ultimately leading to apoptotic cell death [4, 8, 31, 39, 51, 59]. Therefore, further promotion of ROS production by adjuvant agents could be a promising strategy for radiosensitization of cancer cells.

However, due to their higher metabolic rate and dysfunction of mitochondrial oxidative phosphorylation, cancer cells are in a state of elevated oxidative stress and therefore equipped with several enzymatic and non-enzymatic antioxidant defense systems to counteract ROS assault and oxidative injury, maintain a stable redox status, suppress apoptotic death and promote growth [8, 31, 51, 59, 60]. The transcription factor nuclear factor erythroid 2-related factor 2 (Nrf2) is identified as a unique mediator of cellular adaptation to redox stress. This regulator molecule is aberrantly upregulated in many types of cancer cells [8, 31]. In normal conditions, Nrf2 remains at a stable level in the cytoplasm under control of its negative regulator Kelch-like ECH-associated protein 1 (Keap1), forming an inactive complex. However, when exposed to oxidative stress, Nrf2 escapes from its anchor protein Keap1 with subsequent translocation to the nucleus, where it binds to the antioxidant response element (ARE) and regulates the expression of several antioxidant enzyme genes, such as heme oxygenase-1 (HO1), catalase (CAT), superoxide dismutase (SOD), glutathione S-transferase (GST) and NAD(P)H quinone oxidoreductase-1 (NQO1) [8, 31]. These antioxidant mechanisms confer survival of cancer cells under oxidative stress conditions and favor also development of radioresistance phenotype [8, 59]. As expression levels of Nrf2 and many antioxidant enzymes have been shown to be increased in response to radiotherapy, targeting Nrf2-Keap1-ARE signaling pathway and inhibition of Nrf2-dependent antioxidant defense machinery might increase the sensitivity of cancer cells to radiotherapeutic treatment [6, 31, 59] (Figure 2). Accordingly, disturbance of redox status may provide a potential strategy to circumvent radioresistance phenomenon in malignant cells.

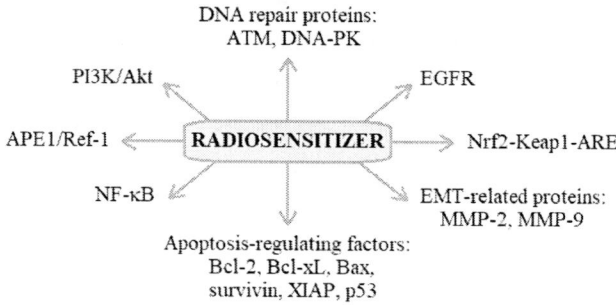

Figure 2. Some potential cellular targets for novel radiosensitizers.

2.2. DNA Damage Signaling

As DNA contains genetic information that is crucial for cellular functioning, DNA damage and genotoxic stress are focal targets of radiotherapy [6, 27, 53]. Therefore, cell killing of ionizing radiation is principally associated with its ability to induce various DNA lesions, including double-strand breaks (DSBs) [3, 15, 16, 19]. Several cellular processes can be initiated in response to radiation-induced DNA damage determining the ultimate fate of the cell, such as initiation of DNA repair mechanisms, modulation of cell cycle progression and induction of apoptotic death [16] (Figure 1). The extent of DNA damage can be characterized by phosphorylation of histone protein H2AX (γ-H2AX) that forms micronuclear foci at the sites of DSBs. γ-H2AX is not only a marker for radiation-induced DSB lesions, but reflects also the level of DNA repair activities [3, 15, 16, 61].

In response to ionizing radiation, the injured cells activate their DNA repair machinery, including DNA-dependent protein kinase (DNA-PK) and ataxia telangiectasia mutated (ATM), to decrease the extent of radiation-induced damage [48]. There are two common cellular mechanisms to repair DNA DSBs: the homologous recombination (HRR) and non-homologous end-joining (NHEJ). These pathways augment DNA repair capacity, facilitate escape of cancer cells from irradiation-induced damage and confer acquiring a radioresistant phenotype [6, 53, 61]. For instance, elevated HRR and NHEJ pathways have been described in radioresistant prostate cancer cells [53]. As responsiveness to radiation therapy is highly dependent on the ability and efficiency of tumor cells to repair radiation-induced DNA damages, most of the current radiosensitization approaches aim to suppress DNA repair capacity and target elements of DNA damage response, such as inhibition of ATM kinase or DNA-PK, to improve radiotherapeutic efficacy and promote cellular apoptosis [3, 6, 15, 38, 61, 62] (Figure 2).

Irradiation-induced genotoxic stress can intervene in cell cycle progression mainly at two checkpoints: G1/S and G2/M phase transitions. These checkpoints are responsive for the genomic instability of malignant cells and control their radiosensitivity [48, 53]. In general, cells at the G2/M phase of the cell cycle are most susceptible to radiation-induced killing, whereas cells in the terminal part of the S phase are least sensitive to ionizing radiation [5, 11, 17, 32, 55].

2.3. APOPTOTIC SIGNALING

The programmed cell death or apoptosis is the primary mode of cell death induced by ionizing radiation in various tumor types and the most desired outcome of cancer radiotherapy [6, 49, 63]. Thus, the efficiency of radiation treatment is related to the intrinsic propensity of malignant cells to undergo apoptosis [62] (Figure 1).

Apoptosis is the normal physiological process that preserves homeostasis and maintains the stability of the intracellular environment. Dysregulation of this process is common in malignancies leading to accumulation of abnormal mutated cells [12, 63, 64]. In general, apoptotic cells are characterized by profound structural and morphological changes, such as a rapid blebbing of the plasma membrane and nuclear collapse associated with DNA cleavage into fragments [49, 63, 64]. Apoptosis can be conducted through two principal signaling mechanisms: death receptor-mediated extrinsic pathway and intrinsic mitochondrial pathway. The latter route has been considered as the primary mode mediating ionizing radiation-induced apoptosis [6, 12, 13]. It is controlled by intracellular prosurvival (Bcl-2, Bcl-xL) and proapoptotic proteins (Bax), which regulate the release of cytochrome c from mitochondria into the cytosol, followed by activation of caspase-9 and caspase-3 and cleavage of PARP [4, 61, 65, 66]. The balance between pro- and antiapoptotic factors is critical in determining the fate of the cell. In particular, a decrease in the Bcl-2 and Bcl-xL proteins is related to genotoxic stress-induced apoptosis, whereas their overexpression enhances cell survival by suppressing apoptotic death [6, 11, 66, 67]. More importantly, elevated levels of prosurvival factors contribute to development of radioresistant phenotype and poor clinical outcome in different types of malignancies [6]. Studies have shown that ionizing radiation can induce the expression of antiapoptotic Bcl-xL in non-small cell lung cancer cells and suppression of Bcl-xL pathway could enhance sensitivity of lung cancer patients to radiotherapy [46]. The overexpression of Bcl-2 induces radioresistance in prostate cancer cells and its repression can lead to overcoming of radioresistant phenotype [48]. Overexpression of Bcl-2 and Bcl-xL proteins confers acquired radioresistance also in human pancreatic cancer cells [6]. Therefore, inhibition of the antiapoptotic functions of Bcl-2 and Bcl-xL and augmentation of proapoptotic action of Bax represent an appealing strategy to combat resistance to radiation therapy.

Another intrinsic cellular mode for apoptotic blockade involves the family of inhibitors of apoptosis protein (IAPs) which inhibit functioning of caspases. Members of this family, such as XIAP and survivin, are frequently overexpressed in tumor cells and contribute to radioresistance, providing potential further targets for development of novel radiosensitizers [6]. Survivin is absent in differentiated normal tissues, but is highly expressed in many malignant cells. Its upregulated levels have been clinically related to radioresistance, disease recurrence and poor overall survival, highlighting the need to develop efficient approaches to counteract this protein [36, 55]. For instance, high expression of survivin has been proposed as one of the predictors for radioresistance in glioblastomas, associated with disease progression and adverse clinical prognosis [42]. Deregulated levels of survivin confer radiotherapy resistance also in breast cancer cells [39]. Upregulation of another member of IAP family, XIAP, has been associated with resistance to radiation-induced cell death in different tumor types [57].

In addition, tumor suppressor protein p53 plays a pivotal role in apoptosis induction [6, 11, 61]. However, p53 gene is mutated in more than 50% of human cancers, whereas its functional mutations lead to enhanced resistance to radiotherapy and worse prognosis in several malignancies [6, 26, 38, 50]. Therefore, it is crucial to improve radiosensitivity also in p53-mutant cancerous cells. Altogether, multiple prosurvival factors governing the inhibition of apoptotic death are usually enhanced in radioresistant tumor cells, whereas agents which promote proapoptotic proteins and increase the rate of apoptosis could act as potentially efficient radiosensitizers [6, 27] (Figure 2).

2.4. Cellular Survival Signaling

One reason for reduction of radiotherapeutic efficacy and development of radioresistance phenotype in malignant cells is the activation of different prosurvival and mitogenic pathways in order to counteract ionizing radiation-induced stress [12, 45, 57]. Exposure of tumor cells to radiation is known to initiate ERK1/2, Akt, NF-κB, STAT3 and COX-2 signaling pathways, promoting the invasive and metastatic character of some cancer cells and accelerating the repopulation of neoplasm [14, 17, 45]. Therefore, targeting these molecular entities and the respective pathways can open new attractive possibilities to intervene in radioresistance and improve therapeutic outcome (Figure 2).

2.4.1. RTK Pathway

One of the most important pathways activated in tumor cells after exposure to ionizing radiation and contributing to the development of radioresistant phenotype is the receptor tyrosine kinase (RTK) signaling [6]. Among RTKs, epidermal growth factor receptor (EGFR) plays an important role in upregulation of prosurvival signaling mechanisms in response to cellular stress, whereas tumors with elevated EGFR expression are usually more radioresistant than tumors with low EGFR levels [6, 48, 57, 68]. The EGFR pathway is triggered via its phosphorylation at tyrosine residues and autophosphorylation of EGFR by radiation induces activation of downstream prosurvival pathways, including ERK1/2, PI3K/Akt and STAT3 [6, 57, 69]. Therefore, agents that target EGFR or its downstream mediators might be efficient radiosensitizers. Previous studies have indeed shown that inhibition of EGFR could contribute to enhanced susceptibility to radiotherapy and apoptotic death in glioma and childhood ependymoma xenografts [6].

2.4.2. PI3K/Akt Pathway

A critical event that facilitates the development of cancer radioresistance is the aberrantly activated protein kinase B (Akt) signaling [19, 70]. Phosphatidylinositol 3-kinase (PI3K)/Akt pathway is a major driving force behind survival, proliferation, growth, metastasis and radiosensitivity of tumor cells, favoring the antiapoptotic environment [5, 6, 19, 35, 55, 71]. Such control over cellular functions is achieved by regulating several important downstream genes, including Bax, Bcl-2, Bcl-xL, Mcl-1 and GLUT-1 [35, 54, 71]. PTEN, a negative regulator of the PI3K/Akt pathway, is often disrupted in diverse tumor tissues [6, 71].

Ionizing radiation-induced DNA damage causes compensatory activation of Akt that fuels survival machinery and protects malignant cells from treatment-induced death, thereby leading to development of radioresistant phenotype [6, 35, 68, 71]. Hence, Akt can be considered as a candidate target to promote radiosensitization and suppression of this signaling cascade could improve the treatment outcome. Inhibition of PI3K/Akt pathway has been indeed described to enhance radiotherapeutic efficacy in several human tumors, such as breast cancer cells [55].

2.4.3. NF-κB Pathway

Nuclear factor-κB (NF-κB) is a major transcription factor that is involved in the control and regulation of cellular proliferation, survival and apoptosis, promoting malignant behavior and tumor progression [16, 20, 72, 73]. In response to ionizing radiation-induced stress, activation of NF-κB pathway promotes the synthesis of downstream molecules that are critical for cell survival and disease progression, and facilitate radioresistance and tumor recurrence in various types of malignancies.

Such downstream targets include several antiapoptotic (Bcl-2, Bcl-xL, XIAP, survivin), proinflammatory (COX-2), proangiogenic (VEGF) and metastatic factors [6, 20, 21, 39, 47, 67]. Overexpression of NF-κB has been suggested to be a good predictor for radioresistance in different tumors, such as in muscle invasive breast cancer [39].

The DNA binding activity of NF-κB is redox-regulated by apurinic/apyrimidinic endonuclease 1/redox factor-1 (APE1/Ref-1) protein [21, 73]. Expression levels of APE1/Ref-1 have been shown to be substantially increased in various tumor tissues, including prostate cancer, after exposure of cells to ionizing radiation, contributing to promotion of resistance to radiotherapy [16, 21, 72]. Reduction of APE1/Ref-1 expression has been correlated with elevated radiosensitivity of tumor cells [21]. Another important transcription factor upregulated by APE1/Ref-1, hypoxia inducible factor-1α (HIF-1α), is involved in cellular survival response to hypoxic environment and is also implicated in radioresistant phenotype [16, 23, 72]. In addition to functioning as a redox activator of diverse transcription factors, such as NF-κB and HIF-1α, APE1/Ref-1 is involved also in DNA repair processes [21, 23, 25, 72]. Therefore, selective targeting of APE1/Ref-1 and suppression of downstream NF-κB signaling pathway could potentiate the response of tumor cells to radiotherapy.

2.4.4. Other Major Processes

Apart from the above-described mechanisms, other cellular events can also contribute to the development of radioresistance, including angiogenesis and increased epithelial-mesenchymal transition (EMT).

Ionizing radiation is known to turn on the angiogenic switch, inducing alterations in endothelial cells and stimulating secretion of proangiogenic molecules, such as vascular endothelial growth factor (VEGF) or nitric oxide synthase (NOS), in different tumor cells [45].

These responses allow malignant cells to survive and negate radiotherapy-induced toxicities [45].

Irradiation can also induce EMT phenomenon in various types of cancerous cells. Exposure to ionizing radiation leads to the transition of cellular morphology more characteristic to mesenchymal phenotype associated with the loss of stable intercellular junctions and decrease in adhesion molecule E-cadherin [27, 28, 33]. EMT is mediated via matrix metalloproteinases (MMPs), especially MMP-2 and MMP-9, which are involved in extracellular matrix degradation and make tumor cells more motile [12, 74]. Thus, EMT is one of the major steps of tumor metastasis accompanied with increased invasion, migration and resistance to radiotherapy, thereby promoting tumor relapse [33, 74]. Several studies have demonstrated that EMT process is regulated by Notch signaling that is activated under irradiation; blocking of this pathway attenuates EMT [27, 28, 33].

Besides apoptosis, autophagy also plays an important role in ionizing radiation-induced tumor cell killing. However, autophagy can exert opposing effects in response to irradiation being either cytoprotective or cytotoxic depending on the radiation dose and biological context [46].

Therefore, combining radiotherapy with agents with antiangiogenic, antiinvasive or antimetastatic properties could improve the efficacy of this important anticancer treatment modality (Figure 2).

Chapter 3

PLANT FLAVONOIDS AS POTENTIAL DIETARY RADIOSENSITIZERS

A substantial body of evidence supports the idea that dietary choices could influence the development, progression, metastasis and mortality of malignant disorders [16, 73, 75]. Current dietary guidelines to fight against cancerous diseases recommend increasing consumption of plant-derived food items [12]. Numerous research findings have indeed shown that various herbs and plant-based products are able to attenuate, retard or reverse the onset of neoplastic processes, but could also serve as therapeutic agents. At that, an important advantage of natural drugs over the conventional treatment modalities is their almost negligible toxicity to normal tissues [4, 6, 12, 13, 16, 44, 63].

Utilization of dietary agents as an adjuvant therapy for traditional treatment modalities is a new attractive area [73]. Emerging evidence suggests that food phytochemicals could be used to potentiate the response of cancer cells to radiotherapy resulting in more killing of tumoral cells than with monotreatment, by modifying different cell survival pathways. Meanwhile, plant compounds can also reduce the radiation-induced toxicity to normal surrounding tissues exposed to radiation beams [14, 15, 65, 73]. Such selective radiosensitization could be achieved by acting through various molecular mechanisms. When combined with ionizing radiation, naturally occurring compounds can suppress the DNA repair efficacy, thereby increasing the extent of genotoxic damage to malignant cells. Phytochemicals are also able to inhibit radiation-induced activation of cellular prosurvival pathways, including RTK, PI3K/Akt and NF-κB signaling, and promote apoptotic death [6]. In addition, plant substances could modulate the redox balance of cancerous cells [6]. It is well known that dietary phytochemicals usually function as strong antioxidants, scavenging free radicals and protecting normal tissues from radiation-induced toxicity, but potentially decreasing also the radiotherapeutic efficacy in cancerous cells [6, 76]. However, under certain conditions, these compounds can paradoxically exhibit prooxidant properties, elevate intracellular ROS level and increase the oxidative damage to tumoral tissues [8, 31, 44, 59, 66]. The redox behavior of plant-derived compounds, i.e., antioxidant vs prooxidant, is determined by several factors, including concentrations, solubility and chelating properties, environmental pH and hypoxia, as well as the presence of metal ions [6, 8, 49, 59]. Therefore, diverse cellular activities might contribute to radiomodulating action of phytochemicals. Accordingly, considerable attention has been recently focused on identification and introduction of novel naturally occurring plant-derived radiosensitizers to augment radiation therapy, overcome radioresistance and achieve improved treatment outcome for various human cancer types [12, 13, 77].

Plant-derived polyphenols, the largest category of phytochemicals, have been used for thousands of years due to their alleged medicinal properties and confirmed biological safety. However, plant phenolics have only recently received significant scientific attention for their ability to modulate various signaling pathways in multistage carcinogenesis process and sensitize tumor cells to traditional anticancer treatment modalities [70]. Flavonoids are a diverse class of plant polyphenols accounting for approximately two-thirds of dietary phenolics (Figure 3).

These compounds are characterized by their diphenylpropane structure (C6-C3-C6) and comprise several groups of agents, such as isoflavones, flavanols, flavonols, flavones, flavanones and anthocyanidins [4, 18]. Flavonoids can be widely found in fruits, vegetables, nuts, seeds and medicinal plants, and are known by their different chemopreventive and chemotherapeutic activities, including antioxidant, antiviral, antibacterial, antiinflammatory, antiangiogenic, antiproliferative, antiinvasive and proapoptotic effects [15, 27, 28, 31, 37, 50]. Although flavonoids are generally not potent enough to be applied as monotherapy in the management of human cancers, these agents can provide a substantial clinical benefit when used in combination with ionizing radiation, sensitizing tumoral cells to radiotherapy while protecting normal tissues from radiation-induced toxicity [16, 18, 31, 50].

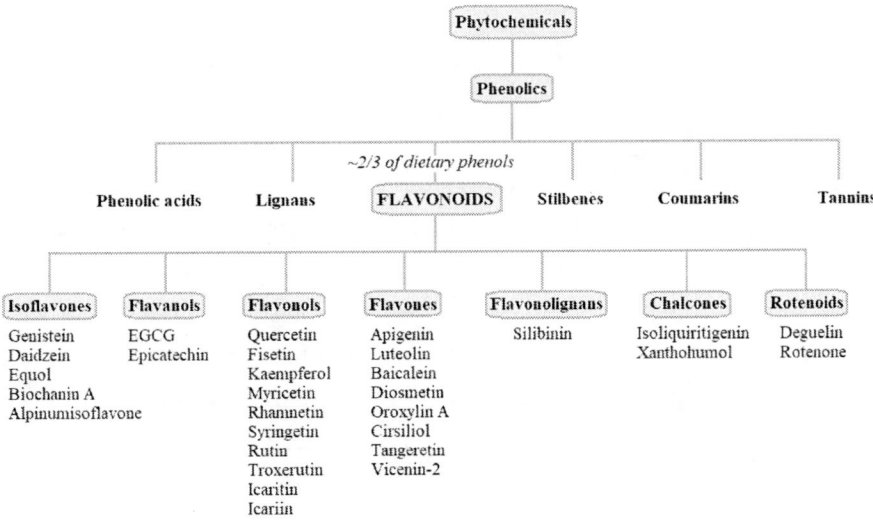

Figure 3. Flavonoids as the largest class of plant phenolics. Their classification and major representatives.

Although structurally diverse flavonoids are ubiquitous in plants, their two most remarkable natural sources in the human diet are probably soybeans and green tea. Soybeans contain plenty of isoflavones, mainly genistein and daidzein, which are metabolically converted to further bioactive derivatives, such as equol [16, 23, 72, 73, 75]. Different isoflavone-rich extracts, such as Novasoy, are currently available also as dietary supplements. As people from Asian countries consume on an average of 10-70 mg soy isoflavones per day, the daily intake in Western populations is only around 1 mg [16, 73, 75]. High levels of soy isoflavones and their metabolites in different body fluids of Asian men have been correlated with lower incidence of prostate cancer [16, 78]. Tea is the most popular beverage in the world with several reported health benefits for humans. Green tea is used as a medicinal agent in Asian region already for more than 4000 years [70]. This popular beverage is the common source of structurally diverse flavanols or catechins, especially epigallocatechin 3-gallate (EGCG) constituting 10-15% of tea polyphenols, but also epigallocatechin, epicatechin 3-gallate, epicatechin and catechin [56, 63, 64, 67]. Concentrated forms of green tea extracts can be found as natural supplements in pharmacies and health food stores. Based on epidemiological studies, consumption of green tea can be inversely associated with breast cancer risk in Asian American and Chinese women [67]. Studies of genistein and EGCG, but also other flavonoids from different subclasses, as potential sensitizers of tumor cells to ionizing radiation have shown promising results in different models of human malignancies and certainly deserve more focus.

Chapter 4

MODULATION OF RADIOTHERAPEUTIC EFFICACY BY DIETARY FLAVONOIDS

4.1. ISOFLAVONES

4.1.1. Genistein, Daidzein, Soy Isoflavones

Genistein is the major and most bioactive isoflavone found in soybeans, daidzein is the second main isoflavone component in soy [20, 72, 79] (Table 1). Regular dietary intake of soy and soy products results in nanomolar plasma concentrations of genistein with reported physiological levels in the range of 276 nM to 6 µM, depending on the isoflavone source and the study subjects [16, 35, 80]. Blood concentrations up to 15 µM have been achieved in human volunteers who consumed 50 mg isoflavones consisting of 40 mg of genistein and daidzein [16, 79, 81]. After ingestion and absorption, genistein distributes throughout the body with relatively high levels in the liver and reproductive organs [36]. Administration of soy isoflavones at low doses has proven to be safe in humans [22].

Table 1. Chemical structures and natural sources of flavonoids

Flavonoid	Chemical structure	Natural sources
ISOFLAVONES		
Daidzein		Soybeans
Genistein		Soybeans
Equol (*isoflavandiol; daidzein metabolite*)		Soybeans
Biochanin A (*methylated isoflavone*)		Red clover (*Trifolium pratense* L.)
Alpinumisoflavone (*pyranoisoflavone*)		*Derris eriocarpa* F.C.How
FLAVANOLS		
Epicatechin		Cocoa, green tea
Epigallocatechin 3-gallate		Green tea

Flavonoid	Chemical structure	Natural sources
FLAVONOLS		
Fisetin		Wide range of plants, fruits and vegetables
Kaempferol		Tea, broccoli, grapefruit, Brussels sprouts, apples
Myricetin		Tea, berries, fruits, vegetables, medicinal herbs
Quercetin		Various vegetables and fruits, such as apples, onions, tomatoes, cauliflower, cabbage; berries, nuts, and Chinese herbal medicines
Rhamnetin (*methylated flavonol*)		Fruits and vegetables; cloves
Syringetin (*methylated flavonol*)		Red grapes and red wine. Isolated from the underground parts of *Achlys triphylla* Smith in A. Rees
Icaritin (*prenylated flavonol*)		Genus *Epimedium*

Table 1. (Continued)

Flavonoid	Chemical structure	Natural sources
Icariin (*prenylated flavonol glycoside*)		Genus *Epimedium*
Rutin (*flavonol glycoside*)		Many plants, fruits, vegetables. Buckwheat, citrus fruits (orange, grapefruit, lemon, lime), berries (mulberry, ash tree fruits, cranberries)
Troxerutin (*flavonol glycoside*)		Tea, coffee, cereal grains, fruits, vegetables
FLAVONES		
Apigenin		Various fruits, vegetables (particularly celery), beans and tea
Baicalein		Root of *Scutellaria baicalensis* Georgi

Flavonoid	Chemical structure	Natural sources
Luteolin		Various fruits and vegetables, including celery, green pepper, perilla leaf, chamomile tea; perilla seeds
Diosmetin (*methylated flavone*)		Olive leaves, citrus fruits, some medicinal herbs
Oroxylin A (*methylated flavone*)		Root of *Scutellaria baicalensis* Georgi
Cirsiliol (*methylated flavone*)		*Achillea fragrantissima* (Forssk.) Sch.Bip., *Salvia guaranitica* A.St.-Hil. Ex Benth.
Tangeretin (*methylated flavone*)		Peel of citrus fruits
Vicenin-2 (*flavone glycoside*)		*Ocimum sanctum* L.
FLAVONOLIGNANS		
Silibinin		Milk thistle (*Silybum marianum* (L.) Gaertn.)

Table 1. (Continued)

Flavonoid	Chemical structure	Natural sources
CHALCONES		
Isoliquiritigenin		Licorice, shallots, bean sprouts
Xanthohumol (*prenylated chalcone*)		Hop plant (*Humulus lupulus* L.)
ROTENOIDS		
Deguelin		*Mundulea sericea* (Willd.) A.Chev.
Rotenone		Tropical and subtropical plant species, especially those of *Lonchocarpus* and *Derris* genera

4.1.1.1. Prostate Cancer

Prostate cancer is the second most common malignant tumor in men, with an estimated 1 276 106 new cases in 2018 worldwide [1]. With continuous aging of the population, the number of patients with clinically diagnosed prostate cancer is expected to increase, representing a growing public health concern. Depending on the disease aggressiveness, radiotherapy can be used either alone or in combination with radical prostatectomy or androgen deprivation therapy for clinical management of localized prostate tumors [24, 76].

The combination of low doses of photon or neutron radiation with genistein at physiologically attainable concentration (15 µM) was shown to suppress DNA synthesis, cell growth and colony formation in PC-3 human prostate carcinoma cells more pronouncedly than irradiation or genistein treatment alone. Such potentiating effect of radiation was achieved by pretreating the cells with genistein for 24 h before irradiation and continuing the incubation in the presence of genistein after radiation for the duration of the experiment, i.e., for 3 days to assess the short-term effects by counting of viable cells and for 10 days for the long-term effects determined by clonogenic assay. Continuous exposure to genistein before and after irradiation was necessary for an optimal response of the cells to combined treatment, as removal of genistein from incubation medium after irradiation lowered the inhibitory effects on colony formation [80] (Table 2). Moreover, pretreatment of PC-3 cells with genistein for 24 h before photon irradiation showed a greater suppression of cell growth than the reverse sequence of radiation followed by genistein 24 h later. Radiation-induced activation of NF-κB was completely inhibited by genistein pretreatment, leading to alterations in expression of regulatory cell cycle proteins, such as upregulation of nuclear $p21^{WAF1/Cip1}$ and downregulation of cyclin B1, thereby stimulating the G2/M phase arrest of cell cycle progression. Promotion of apoptosis was further detected by significantly elevated PARP cleavage [20]. Combined treatment was also shown to suppress the expression of antiapoptotic proteins Bcl-xL and survivin, and promote proapoptotic Bax, suggesting activation of apoptosis-eliciting caspases [82]. Activation of apoptotic machinery was probably initiated by inhibition of radiation-induced APE1/Ref-1 expression by pretreatment of cells with genistein, impairing radiation-induced transcriptional activity of NF-κB and HIF-1α and triggering diverse downstream events ultimately leading to cell death [21, 72].

Table 2. Effects of isoflavones on cancer radiotherapeutic efficacy

Agent	Cancer site	Biological system	Method	Assay conditions	Effect		Ref.
Alpinum-isoflavone, AI	Esophagus	KYSE30 human esophageal squamous cell cancer cells	CCK-8, colony formation	Pretreatment with AI (5 μM) for 24h before irradiation (4, 6 Gy)	↑	Decrease in cell survival. Increase in DNA damage, G2/M arrest and apoptosis. Enhancement of oxidative stress through suppression of Nrf2 and downstream HO1, NQO1	[31]
		Eca109 human esophageal squamous cell cancer cells		Pretreatment with AI (5 μM) for 24h before irradiation (4, 6 Gy)	↑	Decrease in cell survival. Increase in DNA damage, G2/M arrest and apoptosis. Enhancement of oxidative stress through suppression of Nrf2 and downstream HO1, NQO1	[31]
		s.c. injection of Eca109 cells into the right leg of male BALB/c nude mice	Tumor growth analysis	Treatment with AI (20 mg/kg/day); irradiation (6 Gy) on day 10	↑	Regression of tumor, decrease in tumor weight	[31]
Biochanin A, BCA	Colon	HT29 human colon cancer cells	MTT	Pretreatment with BCA (5-100 μM) for 1h before γ-irradiation (2 Gy); incubation for 48h	↑	Decrease in proliferation. Increase in ROS and apoptosis (increase in lipid peroxidation, mitochondrial membrane potential and caspase-3)	[44]
Daidzein, DAI	Cervix	CaSki human cervical cancer cells (high-risk HPV)	Colony formation	Pretreatment with DAI (2.5-40 μM) for 48h before photon irradiation (2, 5, 8 Gy)	~	No effect on radiosensitivity	[35]
		ME180 human cervical cancer cells (HPV39-positive)		Pretreatment with DAI (2.5-40 μM) for 48h before photon irradiation (2, 5, 8 Gy)	~	No effect on radiosensitivity	[35]

Agent	Cancer site	Biological system	Method	Assay conditions	Effect		Ref.
	Prostate	C4-2B human prostate cancer cells (AR-positive, non-responsive to androgen)	Colony formation	Pretreatment with DAI (10 µM) for 48h before photon irradiation (3 Gy); incubation in the presence of DAI in colony assay	↑	Decrease in cell survival. Inhibition of radiation-induced activation of HIF-1α, APE1/Ref-1 and NF-κB	[23]
		PC-3 human prostate cancer cells (AR-negative, non-responsive to androgen)	Colony formation	Pretreatment with DAI (60 µM) for 24h before photon irradiation (3 Gy); incubation in the presence of DAI in colony assay	↑	Decrease in cell survival. Inhibition of radiation-induced activation of HIF-1α, APE1/Ref-1 and NF-κB	[23]
		Injection of PC-3/P1 cells into the prostate of male Balb/c nu/nu nude mice	Tumor growth analysis	Treatment with oral DAI (0.21 mg/day) on days 8-10, irradiation on day 11 (5 Gy), resuming DAI treatment for duration of assay	↑	Inhibition of tumor growth and metastasis to lymph nodes	[23]
Equol, EQ	Breast	MDA-MB-231 human breast cancer cells (basal-like, high-grade, ERα-negative)	Colony formation	Pretreatment with EQ (50 µM) for 72h before X-ray irradiation (6 Gy)	↑	Decrease in survival. Increase in radiation-induced DNA damage and apoptosis	[75]
		T47D human breast cancer cells (poorly or non-invasive; ERα-positive, moderate amount of ERβ)		Pretreatment with EQ (50 µM) for 24h before X-ray irradiation (2, 6 Gy)	↑	Decrease in survival. Increase in radiation-induced apoptosis	[75]
Genistein, GEN	Blood	K562 human myeloid leukemia cells	Counting	Pretreatment with GEN (50 µM) for 1h before γ-irradiation (5 Gy)	↑	Augmentation of death, promotion of cell cycle arrest	[86]
		K562 human chronic myelogenous leukemia cells	Colony formation	Addition of GEN (25 µM) to X-ray irradiated cells (0.1-12 Gy), incubation for 2 weeks	→	Increase in survival, maintenance of G2 arrest, inhibition of radiation-induced death (blocking caspase-3 activity)	[87]

Table 2. (Continued)

Agent	Cancer site	Biological system	Method	Assay conditions	Effect	Ref.
		K562 human chronic myelogenous leukemia cells	Counting	Treatment with GEN (25 µM) and X-ray irradiation (10 Gy)	↓	Prevention of radiation-induced cell death, decrease in nuclear fragmentation. Increase in TK1 expression and activity, maintenance of G2 arrest	[52]
	Brain	U87MG human glioblastoma multiforme cells	MTT, colony formation	Pretreatment with GEN (10, 50 µM) for 30h before γ-irradiation (2 Gy; as single dose or fractionated)	↓↑	Increase in cell survival at 10 µM GEN; reduction of cell survival at 50 µM GEN	[77]
	Breast	MDA-MB-231 human breast cancer cells	Colony formation	Pretreatment with GEN (15 µM) for 24h before photon irradiation (3 Gy); incubation in the presence of GEN in colony assay	↑	Inhibition of colony formation	[20]
		MDA-MB-231 human breast cancer cells (ER-negative)		Pretreatment with GEN (5, 10, 20 µM) for 24h before X-ray irradiation (4 Gy)	↑	Decrease in survival fraction, exacerbation of DNA damage, inhibition of DNA repair. Increase in G2/M arrest and apoptosis (decrease in Bcl-2/Bax ratio)	[11]
		MCF-7 human breast cancer cells (ER-positive)		Pretreatment with GEN (5, 10, 20 µM) for 24h before X-ray irradiation (4 Gy)	↑	Decrease in survival fraction, exacerbation of DNA damage, inhibition of DNA repair. Increase in G2/M arrest and apoptosis (decrease in Bcl-2/Bax ratio)	[11]
	Cervix	CaSki human cervical cancer cells (high-risk HPV)	Colony formation	Pretreatment with GEN (2.5-40 µM) for 48h before photon irradiation (5, 8 Gy)	↑	Reduction of colony formation. Decrease in Mcl-1 and pAkt	[35]

Agent	Cancer site	Biological system	Method	Assay conditions	Effect		Ref.
		CaSki human cervical cancer cells (HPV16-positive)	MTT	Pretreatment with GEN (200 μM) for 1h before γ-irradiation (10 Gy)	↑	Decrease in cell viability. Increase in G2/M arrest and apoptosis (cyt c release, decrease in Bcl-2, increase in Bax, cleavage of caspases-3/-8). Downregulation of E6 and E7 levels; increase in ROS; inhibition of radiation-induced COX-2 expression and PGE2 production	[66]
		HeLa human cervical adenocarcinoma cells		Pretreatment with GEN (40, 100 μM) for 48h before γ-irradiation (4 Gy)	↑	Inhibition of proliferation. Increase in G2/M arrest and apoptosis. Decrease in radiation-induced survivin expression	[36]
		ME180 human cervical cancer cells (HPV39-positive)	Colony formation	Pretreatment with GEN (20, 40 μM) for 48h before photon irradiation (2, 5, 8 Gy)	↑	Reduction of colony formation. Increase in G2/M arrest, decrease in Mcl-1 and pAkt	[35]
	Colorectum	HCT116 human colorectal cancer cells	Colony formation	Pretreatment with GEN (10, 50, 100 μM) for 24h before photon irradiation (1, 2, 4 Gy)	↓~	Weakly antagonistic or additive antiproliferative effects. Very weak reduction of EGFR phosphorylation, upregulation of activated AKT and ERK1/2	[68]
	Esophagus	TE-1 human esophageal squamous cell cancer cells (p53-mutant)	Colony formation	Pretreatment with GEN (30 μM) for 3h before X-ray irradiation (5 Gy), incubation for 6h prior to assay	↑	Reduction of survival fraction. Abolishment of radiation-induced activation of p42/p44 ERK, AKT, decrease in cyclin D1	[69]
		TE-2 human esophageal squamous cell cancer cells (p53 wt)		Pretreatment with GEN (30 μM) for 3h before X-ray irradiation (5 Gy), incubation for 6h prior to assay	↑	Reduction of survival fraction. Abolishment of radiation-induced activation of p42/p44 ERK, AKT, decrease in cyclin D1. Increase in apoptosis (decrease in Bcl-2, increase in Bax, cleavage of PARP)	[69]

Table 2. (Continued)

Agent	Cancer site	Biological system	Method	Assay conditions	Effect		Ref.
	Kidney	RC-2 human renal cell carcinoma cells	Colony formation	Pretreatment with GEN (15 µM) for 24h before photon irradiation (3 Gy); incubation in the presence of GEN in colony assay	↑	Inhibition of colony formation	[20]
		KCI-18 human renal cell carcinoma cells	Colony formation	Pretreatment with GEN (15 µM) for 24h before photon irradiation (3 Gy); incubation in the presence of GEN in colony assay	↑	Inhibition of colony formation	[20]
		Injection of KCI-18 cells in the right kidney of female BALB/C nu/nu nude mice	Tumor growth analysis	Pretreatment with oral GEN (5 mg/day) on days 12-14; irradiation on day 15 (8 Gy); resuming GEN administration every other day for duration of assay	↑	Inhibition of tumor growth and progression	[81]
	Liver	Reuber H35 rat hepatoma cells	Colony formation	Pretreatment with GEN (60, 90, 120 µM) for 30 min before X-ray irradiation (2-8 Gy), continuing incubation for 23.5h	↑	Reduction of survival	[84]
	Lung	A549 human non-small cell lung cancer cells (ERα- and ERβ-positive)	Colony formation	Pretreatment with GEN (0.01, 10 µM) for 24h before X-ray irradiation (2, 4 Gy)	↑~	Reduction of clonogenic survival in A549 with mutated p53; no effect in A549 with wt p53	[26]

Agent	Cancer site	Biological system	Method	Assay conditions	Effect		Ref.
		A549 human non-small cell lung cancer cells	MTT, colony formation	Pretreatment with GEN (10 μM) for 48h before X-ray irradiation (4 Gy)	Inhibition of growth and clonogenic survival. Increase in radiation-induced ROS and oxidative damage, decrease in reduced GSH. Demethylation of Keap1 promoter, decrease in nuclear Nrf2 and downstream NQO1. Increase in radiation-induced apoptosis	↑	[60]
		A549 human non-small cell lung cancer cells	CCK-8	Pretreatment with GEN (30, 60 μM) for 24h before irradiation (2, 4 Gy)	Inhibition of growth. Increase in DNA damage, apoptosis (increase in Bax, cleaved PARP, caspase-3; decrease in Bcl-xL) and autophagy (increase in LC3II, Beclin-1	↑	[46]
		s.c. injection of A549 cells into female nude mice	Tumor growth analysis	i.p. injection of GEN daily (100 mg/kg bw), followed by irradiation for 3 days later (6 Gy)	Synergistic inhibition of tumor growth	↑	[46]
	Prostate	C4-2B human prostate cancer cells (AR-positive, non-responsive to androgen)	Colony formation	Pretreatment with GEN (10 μM) for 48h before photon irradiation (3 Gy); incubation in the presence of GEN in colony assay	Decrease in survival. Inhibition of radiation-induced HIF-1α, APE1/Ref-1 and NF-κB	↑	[23]
		DU145 human prostate cancer cells (androgen-independent)		Pretreatment with GEN (5, 15 μM) for 24h before X-ray irradiation (1, 3, 5 Gy)	Increase in G2/M arrest and apoptosis	↑	[78]
		DU145 human prostate cancer cells	CCK-8	Pretreatment with GEN (30 μM) for 1h before X-ray irradiation (4 Gy); incubation for 24h	Induction of S phase arrest, promotion of apoptosis (increase in ATM, Bax, caspase-3; decrease in p-IGF1R, Bcl-2). Inhibition of DNA repair via inactivation of NHEJ and HRR pathways	↑	[53]

Table 2. (Continued)

Agent	Cancer site	Biological system	Method	Assay conditions	Effect		Ref.
		s.c. injection of DU145 cells in the flank of male nude mice	Tumor growth analysis	Pretreatment with GEN (100 mg/kg/ day) before X-ray irradiation every three days for 5 times	↑	Decrease in proliferation index of tumor volume	[53]
		LNCaP human prostate cancer cells (ERα- and ERβ-positive, androgen-sensitive)	Colony formation	Pretreatment with GEN (10 µM) for 24h before irradiation (0.4-2 Gy); followed by incubation with GEN for 24h	↑	Increase in low-dose HRS. Abolishment of radiation-induced p21 expression	[83]
		PC-3 human prostate carcinoma cells	Counting, colony formation	Pretreatment with GEN (15 µM) for 24h before photon (2, 3 Gy) or neutron (0.5, 1, 1.5 Gy) irradiation; incubation with GEN for 3 days (counting) or 10 days (colony assay)	↑	Inhibition of cell growth, colony formation and DNA synthesis	[80]
		PC-3 human prostate carcinoma cells	Colony formation	Pretreatment with GEN (15 µM) for 24h before photon irradiation (2, 3 Gy); incubation in the presence of GEN in colony assay	↑	Suppression of colony formation. Increase in G2/M arrest (increase in nuclear p21WAF1/Cip1, decrease in cyclin B1) and apoptosis (PARP cleavage). Inhibition of radiation-induced NF-κB activation	[20]
		PC-3 human prostate carcinoma cells		Pretreatment with GEN (30 µM) for 24h before photon irradiation (3 Gy); incubation in the presence of GEN in colony assay	↑	Increase in apoptosis (decrease in Bcl-xL, survivin; increase in Bax, cleaved PARP)	[82]

Agent	Cancer site	Biological system	Method	Assay conditions	Effect		Ref.
		PC-3 human prostate cancer cells	Colony formation	Pretreatment with GEN (15 µM) for 24h before photon irradiation (3 Gy); incubation in the presence of GEN in colony assay	↑	Inhibition of survival, increase in apoptosis. Suppression of radiation-induced APE1/Ref-1 and NF-κB activation	[21]
		PC-3 human prostate cancer cells (ERα- and ERβ-negative, androgen-independent)		Pretreatment with GEN (10 µM) for 24h before irradiation (0.5-2 Gy)	↓	Abolishment of low-dose HRS. Increase in resistance to low irradiation doses	[83]
		PC-3 human prostate cancer cells (AR-negative, non-responsive to androgen)		Pretreatment with GEN (30 µM) for 72h before photon irradiation (3 Gy)	↑	Inhibition of radiation-induced activation of Src/STAT3/HIF-1α pathway. Decrease in APE1/Ref-1, and DNA binding activity of HIF-1α and NF-κB	[72]
		PC-3 human prostate cancer cells (AR-negative, non-responsive to androgen)	Colony formation	Pretreatment with GEN (15 µM) for 24h before photon irradiation (3 Gy); incubation in the presence of GEN in colony assay	↑	Decrease in survival. Inhibition of radiation-induced HIF-1α, APE1/Ref-1 and NF-κB	[23]
		PC-3 human prostate cancer cells	CCK-8	Pretreatment with GEN (30 µM) for 1h before X-ray irradiation (4 Gy); incubation for 24h	↑	Induction of S phase arrest, promotion of apoptosis (increase in ATM, Bax, caspase-3; decrease in p-IGF1R, Bcl-2). Inhibition of DNA repair via inactivation of NHEJ and HRR pathways	[53]

Table 2. (Continued)

Agent	Cancer site	Biological system	Method	Assay conditions	Effect		Ref.
		Implantation of PC-3 cells in the prostate of male Balb/c nu/nu nude mice	Tumor growth analysis	Oral treatment with GEN (5 mg/day) on days 13, 14; photon irradiation on day 15 (5 Gy); resuming GEN administration every other day for duration of assay	↑	Inhibition of tumor growth, decrease in number of enlarged lymph nodes and lymph nodes weight. Increase in mouse survival in long-term treatment with GEN (3 months)	[22]
		Implantation of PC-3 cells in the prostate of male Balb/c nu/nu nude mice	Tumor growth analysis	Oral treatment with GEN (0.43 mg/day) on days 8-10, irradiation on day 11 (5 Gy); resuming GEN administration daily for duration of assay	↑	Inhibition of tumor growth and metastasis to lymph nodes. In situ tissue alterations and tumor destruction	[82]
		Implantation of PC-3/PI cells in the prostate of male Balb/c nu/nu nude mice	Tumor growth analysis	Oral treatment with GEN (0.43 mg/day) on days 8-10; irradiation on day 11 (5 Gy); resuming GEN administration daily for duration of assay	↑	Inhibition of tumor growth. Downregulation of APE1/Ref-1 expression, inhibition of NF-κB activation	[21]
		RM-9 murine prostate cancer cells	Colony formation	Pretreatment with GEN (10, 15 μM) for 24h before γ-irradiation (3 Gy)	↑	Augmentation of growth inhibition	[79]
		Injection of RM-9 cells in the prostate of male C57BL/6 mice	Tumor growth analysis	Pretreatment with GEN (1 mg/day) on days 8-10; irradiation on day 11 (8 Gy); resuming GEN administration every other day for duration of assay	↑	Inhibition of tumor growth, decrease in tumor volume. Suppression of spontaneous metastasis to regional para-aortic lymph nodes	[79]

Agent	Cancer site	Biological system	Method	Assay conditions	Effect		Ref.
	Soft tissue	S180 murine sarcoma cells	Counting	Pretreatment with GEN (10 µM) for 24h before X-ray irradiation (2 Gy)	↑	Decrease in survival fraction, increase in apoptosis (increase in Bax, decrease in Bcl-2, cyt c release). Inhibition of DSB repair via inactivation of DNA-PKcs leading to incompleteness of NHEJ and HR repairs	[61]
		Inoculation of S180 cells in female Balb/c mice	Tumor growth analysis	i.p. injection of GEN (200 mg/kg/ bw) for 24h before fractionated whole-body X-ray irradiation (2 Gy/ fraction for 5 times)	↑	Inhibition of tumor weight and volume. Increase in apoptosis (increase in Bax, decrease in Bcl-2, cyt c release)	[61]
G2535 (GEN 43%, DAI 21%, glycitein 2%)	Prostate	C4-2B human prostate cancer cells (AR-positive, non-responsive to androgen)	Colony formation	Pretreatment with G2535 (10 µM) for 48h before photon irradiation (3 Gy); incubation in the presence of G2535 in colony assay	↑	Decrease in cell survival. Inhibition of radiation-induced activation of HIF-1α, APE1/Ref-1 and NF-κB	[23]
		PC-3 human prostate carcinoma cells		Pretreatment with soy isoflavones (10, 15 µM) for 24h before photon irradiation (3 Gy); incubation with soy isoflavones during colony assay	↑	Decrease in survival, increase in apoptosis (decrease in Bcl-xL, survivin; increase in Bax, cleaved PARP)	[82]
		PC-3 human prostate cancer cells		Pretreatment with soy isoflavones (10, 15 µM) for 24h before photon irradiation (3 Gy); incubation with soy isoflavones during colony assay	↑	Decrease in survival, increase in apoptosis. Inhibition of radiation-induced APE1/Ref-1 and NF-κB activation	[21]

Table 2. (Continued)

Agent	Cancer site	Biological system	Method	Assay conditions	Effect		Ref.
		PC-3 human prostate cancer cells (AR-negative, non-responsive to androgen)		Pretreatment with G2535 (30 µM) for 72h before photon irradiation (3 Gy)	↑	Inhibition of radiation-induced activation of Src/STAT3/HIF-1α pathway. Decrease in APE1/Ref-1, and DNA binding activity of HIF-1α and NF-κB; reduction of VEGF production	[72]
		PC-3 human prostate cancer cells (AR-negative, non-responsive to androgen)	Colony formation	Pretreatment with G2535 (15 µM) for 24h before photon irradiation (3 Gy); incubation in the presence of G2535 in colony assay	↑	Decrease in cell survival. Inhibition of radiation-induced activation of HIF-1α, APE1/Ref-1 and NF-κB	[23]
		Implantation of PC-3 cells in the prostate of male Balb/c nu/nu mice	Tumor growth analysis	Oral treatment with soy isoflavones (1 mg/day) on days 8-10, irradiation on day 11 (5 Gy), resuming daily soy isoflavones treatment for duration of assay	↑	Inhibition of tumor growth and metastasis to lymph nodes. In situ tissue alterations and tumor destruction	[82]
		Injection of PC-3/PI cells in the prostate of male Balb/c nu/nu mice		Oral treatment with soy isoflavones (1 mg/day) on days 8-10, irradiation on day 11 (5 Gy), resuming daily soy isoflavones treatment for duration of assay	↑	Decrease in tumor growth. Downregulation of APE1/Ref-1 expression, inhibition of NF-κB activation	[21]

Agent	Cancer site	Biological system	Method	Assay conditions	Effect		Ref.
G4660 (GEN 83.3%, DAI 14.6%, glycitein 0.26%)		Injection of PC-3/PI cells into the prostate of male Balb/c nu/nu nude mice	Tumor growth analysis	Oral treatment with G2535 (1 mg/day) on days 8-10, irradiation on day 11 (5 Gy), resuming G2535 treatment for duration of assay	↑	Inhibition of tumor growth and metastasis to lymph nodes	[23]
	Lung	A549 human non-small cell lung cancer cells	Colony formation	Pretreatment with G4660 (5, 7.5, 10 µM) for 72h before X-ray irradiation (3 Gy); incubation in the presence of G4660	↑	Synergistic reduction of survival. Augmentation of radiation-induced DNA damage (DSBs); blocking of radiation-induced HIF-1α, APE1/Ref-1 and NF-κB activation	[25]
		H1650 human non-small cell lung cancer cells	Counting	Pretreatment with G4660 (10, 25 µM) for 24h before X-ray irradiation (3 Gy)	↑	Inhibition of cell growth	[25]
		i.v. injection of A549 cells in the tail vein of female Hsd Athymic Nude-Foxn1nu nu/nu nude mice	Tumor growth analysis	Oral treatment with G4660 (1 mg/day) on days 20-22, irradiation to the left lung (12 Gy) on day 22; resuming daily G4660 treatment for 4 weeks	↑	Decrease in cell viability, reduction of tumor nodules	[30]
		i.v. injection of A549 cells in the tail vein of female Hsd Athymic Nude-Foxn1nu nu/nu nude mice		Oral treatment with G4660 (5 mg/day) on days 16-18, irradiation to the thorax on day 19 (10 Gy); resuming G4660 treatment at 5 mg/day for 5 more days, then 1 mg/day for 4 weeks	↑	Inhibition of tumor growth. Increase in areas of lung tissues free of tumor	[29]

Radiosensitizing effect of genistein was observed also in an orthotopic prostate carcinoma model of PC-3 cells in nude mice. Oral pretreatment of established prostate tumors with genistein for 2 days before tumor irradiation followed by resumption of genistein treatment every other day at one day after irradiation for 4 weeks resulted in significantly stronger inhibition of primary tumor growth compared to genistein or radiation alone. The tumors treated in conjunction with radiation and genistein showed reduced expression of proliferation marker Ki-67 and large areas of tumor destruction replaced by fibrotic tissue, inflammatory cells and apoptotic cells. In addition, the number of metastatic para-aortic lymph nodes was also reduced by combined treatment, eventually leading to significantly increased survival of mice in long-term experiments. However, treatment with genistein alone unexpectedly increased (but not decreased) the size and the mean weight of para-aortic lymph nodes due to heavy tumor infiltration, meaning that pure genistein as a single treatment modality could stimulate metastatic spread from the primary tumor site to regional lymph nodes via the lymphatic system [22]. Being of concern regarding intake of genistein by prostate cancer patients, this intriguing finding raised two further questions: first, whether the prometastatic action of genistein can be dependent on immune status of the experimental mice model; and second, do other isoflavones in soy also promote metastatic spread of prostate tumor.

To determine whether the enhancement of metastatic spread by genistein was specific for PC-3 xenograft bearing mice due to their impaired immune system, syngeneic RM-9 orthotopic prostate tumor model in immunocompetent mice was further explored. Genistein pretreatment (10-15 µM) enhanced irradiation-induced decrease in survival fraction of RM-9 murine prostate cancer cells *in vitro*, and led to a greater inhibition of tumor progression and metastasis in mice with implanted RM-9 tumor *in vivo* compared to either modality alone. Large areas of tumor destruction with extensive fibrosis and necrosis and occurrence of apoptotic and inflammatory cells were observed followed to the treatment with genistein and radiation. Also, the mean weight of regional para-aortic lymph nodes was significantly reduced in the mice receiving combined treatment compared to their counterparts treated with radiation alone. However, similarly to human xenotransplant PC-3 orthotopic model, monotreatment of syngeneic RM-9 orthotopic tumor bearing mice with genistein caused an increase in the size of para-aortic lymph nodes, showing that this paradoxical phenomenon was independent on the murine immune status, i.e., immunodeficient vs immunocompetent, or on the mouse strain [79].

To unravel the potential effect of other isoflavones on metastatic spread of prostate tumor, a natural formulation consisting of 43% genistein, 21% daidzein and 2% glycitein, known as G2535, was further studied. Such a mixture is representative of soy isoflavones pills actually used in human interventions. As a result, this mixture of soy isoflavones potentiated radiation-induced cell killing in PC-3 carcinoma cells *in vitro* [21, 82] and sensitized prostate cancer cells to ionizing radiation even more potently than pure genistein [21]. Enhancement of susceptibility to radiation by soy isoflavones was associated with suppression of antiapoptotic proteins Bcl-xL and survivin, promotion of proapoptotic Bax and cleavage of PARP, suggesting activation of apoptotic pathways [82]. Mechanistically, pretreatment with soy isoflavones led to inhibition of radiation-induced nuclear APE1/Ref-1 expression and DNA binding activity of NF-κB and HIF-1α, thereby blocking radiation-induced survival pathways, such as Src/STAT3/HIF-1α, and driving the cells to apoptotic cascades [21, 72]. Potentiation of the radiation effect by soy isoflavones was independent on the status of androgen receptors in prostate tumor cells, as similarly to androgen receptor-negative PC-3 cells, genistein or soy isoflavones enhanced radiation-induced cell killing also in androgen receptor-positive C4-2B human prostate cancer cells [23]. Using the PC-3 orthotopic metastatic model in nude mice, combined treatment with oral soy isoflavones and tumor irradiation resulted in greater inhibition of primary tumor growth and metastasis to lymph nodes compared to either modality alone. Prostate tumors treated with soy isoflavones and radiation revealed *in situ* tissue alterations and large areas of tumor destruction replaced by fibrosis beside appearance of numerous apoptotic and inflammatory cells [21, 82]. Consistent with molecular alterations observed *in vitro*, treatment of established prostate tumors with soy isoflavones and radiation resulted in downregulation of APE1/Ref-1 protein and NF-κB activity, similar to combined treatment with genistein and radiation [21]. However, in contrast to pure genistein, mixture of soy isoflavones as monotreatment did not promote metastatic spread to para-aortic lymph nodes. This discrepancy could be related to the ability of pure genistein, but not soy isoflavones, to induce HIF-1α and hypoxic microenvironment in prostate tumors conferring increased metastasis [82]. It is probable that daidzein in composition of soy isoflavones mixture provided protection against the adverse prometastatic effects of genistein. Pure daidzein acted as a radiosensitizer for prostate tumors in PC-3 and C4-2B cells *in vitro* and in orthotopic PC-3 tumor bearing mice *in vivo*. The effects caused by daidzein on inhibition of radiation-induced APE1/Ref-1, HIF-1α and NF-κB pathways were still somewhat milder than those observed with pure genistein or soy isoflavones mixture. Therefore, in addition to genistein, daidzein as a second bioactive component of soy isoflavones can also contribute to suppression of cell survival cascades activated in response to radiation-induced oxidative and genotoxic stress, resulting in augmentation of radiation-induced cell death [23].

In addition, micromolar doses of genistein (5 μM and 15 μM) enhanced radiation efficacy also in another androgen-independent human prostate cancer cell line, DU145. The mechanism behind this radiosensitizing effect involved prolonged cell cycle arrest in G2/M phase and increased apoptotic death [78]. Somewhat higher doses of genistein (30 μM) potentiated antiproliferative and proapoptotic action of radiation in both DU145 and PC-3 cells, enhancing irradiation-induced DSBs and suppressing DNA repair via inactivation of homologous recombination and non-homologous end joining pathways. Enhancement of radiation efficacy was accompanied by increased levels of ATM, Bax and caspase-3, and reduced expression of Bcl-2 protein. Oral administration of genistein to DU145 tumor bearing mice before treatment with ionizing radiation resulted in significantly reduced proliferation index of tumor volume revealing increased sensitivity to radiotherapy [53].

Furthermore, preincubation with genistein (10 μM) enhanced the low-dose hyper-radiosensitivity (HRS) phenomenon in androgen-sensitive LNCaP human prostate cancer cells when combined with low irradiation doses between 0.4-2 Gy. On the contrary, low-dose HRS was abolished by genistein in androgen-independent PC-3 cells, where genistein increased radioresistance to low irradiation doses. However, as these findings were described only *in vitro* conditions, caution should be exercised with their further interpretation [83].

As a whole, genistein, daidzein and soy isoflavones formulation consisting of genistein, daidzein and glycitein may function as potent radiosensitizers for prostate cancer cells *in vitro*, independent on the status of androgen receptors in tumor cells. Moreover, pretreatment with these natural agents can improve the control of primary tumor growth and suppress spontaneous metastasis to lymph nodes when combined with irradiation of established prostate tumors both in syngeneic as well as xenograft models, revealing relevance for further clinical application to manage locally advanced prostate tumors. Therefore, the design of clinical trials for prostate cancer patients with localized disease is important to improve radiotherapeutic outcome and survival rate in the future. To date, it has been only preliminarily demonstrated that administration of soy isoflavones (Novasoy, 200 mg/day for 6 months) to patients with localized prostate cancer undergoing fractionated radiotherapy (1.8-2.5 Gy fractions for a total dose of 73.8-77.5 Gy) decreased radiation-induced incidence of urinary, intestinal and sexual dysfunction, with no reduction but rather some improvement of radiotherapeutic efficacy [24].

4.1.1.2. Renal Cell Carcinoma

In parallel to increasing prevalence of risk factors in recent years, such as smoking, obesity and hypertension, incidence of renal cell carcinoma has also continuously raised [81]. In 2018, the global number of new kidney cancer cases was estimated to 403 262 [1]. Patients with advanced renal cell carcinoma commonly develop metastases in the lungs, liver and mesentery, which are only poorly responsive to conventional treatment modalities, including radiotherapy [81].

Pretreatment of KCI-18 and RC-2 human renal cell carcinoma cells with genistein (15 µM) for 24 h followed by photon radiation and continued exposure to genistein resulted in a significant potentiation of radiation-induced tumor cell death [20] (Table 2). In orthotopic KCI-18 metastatic xenograft model in athymic nude mice, oral administration of genistein for 3 days before radiation of tumor-bearing kidney caused a greater inhibition of primary tumor growth and control of mesentery metastasis than either modality alone. Histologically, destruction of tumor tissue by combined treatment was accompanied by induction of atypical giant cells. However, treatment of established kidney tumors with genistein as a single therapy demonstrated a tendency to promote the growth of primary kidney tumor and enhance metastatic spread to the mesentery lining of the bowel (but still not distant metastasis to the lungs). Such facilitated migration of tumor cells to proximal organs could occur via adipose tissue blood vessels because of high vascularization of kidney tumors. Although the prometastatic effect of genistein was previously observed also in different orthotopic prostate cancer models, treatment with genistein did still not increase the growth of primary prostate tumors revealing some differences with renal cell carcinoma [81]. Nevertheless, pretreatment with genistein could potentiate radiotherapeutic efficacy in renal cell carcinoma, improving control of both primary tumor growth and metastasis.

4.1.1.3. Non-Small Cell Lung Cancer

Lung cancer is the global leading cause of cancer incidence and mortality in men and women, with an estimated 2 093 876 new cases in 2018 worldwide [1, 74]. About 85% of primary lung cancer patients suffer from non-small cell lung cancer with adenocarcinoma as the most common subtype [25, 29, 62].

Pretreatment of A549 human non-small cell lung cancer cells with physiologically achievable doses of genistein (0.01 µM, 10 µM) was shown to enhance their susceptibility to ionizing radiation. However, such radiosensitizing ability of genistein was essentially dependent on p53 status of A549 cells, occurring only in mutated p53 expressing cells and not in cells with wild-type p53, regardless of higher intrinsic radiosensitivity in wild-type p53 cells. These results show that genistein could specifically sensitize radioresistant clones [26] (Table 2). When combined with radiation, genistein (10 µM) caused a further increase in ROS level, aggravated radiation-induced oxidative stress and oxidative damage in A549 cells, thereby potentiating inhibition of cell growth and clonogenic survival and promoting apoptotic death. Augmentation of apoptosis was characterized by release of cytochrome c from mitochondria to the cytosol and increased cleavage of caspase-3. This radiosensitizing effect was achieved through induction of Keap1 expression by genistein, inhibiting nuclear translocation of Nrf2 and subsequently reducing the levels of target antioxidant enzyme genes. Moreover, potentiation of radiation efficacy was selective for A549 cells and did not appear in normal lung fibroblasts MRC-5, where radiation-induced oxidative stress was rather decreased by genistein, probably resulting from intrinsically different redox status of malignant and normal cells [60]. Pretreatment with somewhat higher doses of genistein (30 µM, 60 µM) before radiation of A549 cells augmented not only radiation-induced apoptotic death but also autophagic death due to suppression of Bcl-xL levels in the cytoplasm and promotion of dissociation of Bcl-xL from Beclin-1. Lower levels of cytoplasmic Bcl-xL were closely related to radiosensitivity of non-small cell lung cancer cells. Combined treatment with genistein and ionizing radiation led to significantly greater inhibition of cell growth and more apoptosis than either treatment alone, characterized by elevated expression of DNA damage marker γ-H2AX, proapoptotic Bax protein, caspase-3 and cleaved PARP in A549 cells. Enhanced level of LC3II protein was indicative of increased autophagy. In addition, treatment of A549 xenograft bearing mice with genistein in conjunction with radiation resulted in a synergistic inhibition of tumor growth [46]. Therefore, the current data are promising concerning application of genistein to enhance radiotherapeutic efficacy in non-small cell lung cancer patients, especially with radioresistant tumors.

Besides pure genistein, the radiosensitizing potential of soy isoflavones mixture, consisting of 83.3% genistein, 14.6% daidzein and 0.26% glycitein, known as G4660, was also explored in human non-small cell lung cancer preclinical models. This formulation is consistent with the soy isoflavones pills used in human interventions in clinical studies and has proven to be safe [25]. G4660 soy isoflavones mixture potentiated radiation-induced killing of A549 cells, increasing formation of DNA double-strand breaks and blocking the DNA repair processes. Mechanisms behind this radiosensitization by soy isoflavones involved inhibition of cellular survival pathways upregulated by radiation, such as suppression of APE1/Ref-1 expression and attenuation of DNA binding activity of transcription factors NF-κB and HIF-1α, driving cells to death cascades. Augmentation of radiation-induced cell killing was observed also in another human non-small cell lung cancer cell line, H1650. As A549 cells express wild-type EGFR and mutant KRAS, while H1650 cells express mutant EGFR and wild-type KRAS, radiosensitization of human non-small cell lung cancer cells by soy isoflavones seems to be independent on their EGFR and KRAS mutation status [25]. Furthermore, oral administration of soy isoflavones to A549 tumor-bearing nude mice followed by treatment with ionizing radiation and continued exposure to soy isoflavones led to decrease in the number of tumor nodules and stronger inhibition of tumor growth compared to either modality alone, resulting in greater areas of lung parenchyma free of tumors [29, 30]. At that, soy isoflavones were more effective for enhancing tumor response to radiotherapy when they were given prior to radiation, with 2.5-fold smaller tumors in mice receiving soy isoflavones 3 days before radiation than in mice receiving soy isoflavones on the day of radiation [29]. Tumor nodules treated with genistein in conjunction with radiation exhibited degenerative changes and extensive inflammatory infiltrates, besides lowered expression of proliferation marker Ki-67 [29, 30]. At the same time, soy isoflavones reduced the extent of radiation-induced injury in normal lung tissue, reducing pneumonitis, fibrosis and protecting bronchioles [29]. These findings highlight the potential use of soy isoflavones as a safe dietary complementary approach to augment radiotherapeutic efficacy, revealing new options for optimizing treatment outcome of lung cancer patients in clinical settings. Considering the possible radioprotective effects of soy isoflavones on normal surrounding tissues, this strategy could be especially attractive for patients with already compromised lung functions.

4.1.1.4. Breast Cancer

Breast cancer is the most common type of malignancy in women with an estimated 2 088 849 new cases in 2018 worldwide, being also the global leading cause of cancer death among females [1]. Increased incidence of breast cancer cases all over the world requires the use of different treatment modalities, including combinations of surgery, chemotherapy, hormonal treatment and radiotherapy [55, 57]. The exact choice of therapy as well as predicted response to treatment of this clinically and molecularly heterogenous disease are largely dependent on the presence of hormone receptors in malignant tissue, i.e., estrogen receptor (ER), progesterone receptor and human epidermal growth factor receptor 2 [11, 75]. ER-negative tumors are generally less susceptible to treatment being related to their worse prognosis [75].

Pretreatment with genistein (15 µM) for 24 h followed by irradiation led to augmentation of radiation-induced cell killing in ER-negative human breast cancer cells MDA-MB-231 [20] (Table 2). Combination of genistein and radiation resulted in greater inhibition of clonogenic survival, exacerbation of DNA damage and suppression of DNA repair compared to either treatment alone in both MDA-MB-231 as well as ER-positive human breast cancer cells MCF-7, showing that radiosensitizing effect of genistein could be independent on ER status of breast tumors. Combined treatment of breast cancer cells with genistein and radiation enhanced remarkably the number of cells at G2/M phase and promoted subsequent apoptotic death, with upregulation of Bax and downregulation of Bcl-2 proteins [11]. Therefore, instead of the direct cytotoxic action by itself, genistein obviously potentiates the radiosensitivity of molecularly different types of breast cancer cells.

4.1.1.5. Cervical Cancer

Cervical cancer represents 6.6% of global cancer incidence in women, with an estimated 569 847 new cases in 2018 worldwide [1]. Development of cervical cancer is closely related to infection with human papillomaviruses (HPVs). During malignant progression, the HPV genome commonly integrates into the host DNA, leading to expression of two viral oncoproteins, E6 and E7, which promote degradation of the p53 and pRb tumor suppressor proteins, respectively [66]. The treatment of locally advanced disease by combination of surgical resection and radiotherapy has often remained insufficient [66].

Action of genistein as radiosensitizer for cervical tumor cells was somewhat variable. ME180 human cervical cancer cells (HPV39-positive) were more sensitive to radiation response at genistein (20 µM, 40 µM) than CaSki human cervical cancer cells (high risk HPV16-positive). Differently from ME180 cells, p53 is inactivated by HPVE6 protein in CaSki cells. At 40 μM genistein, even less than 5% of ME180 cells survived the radiation doses 2-8 Gy. Although potentiation of radiation effect in CaSki cells also appeared at 5 and 8 Gy, it was not dependent on genistein doses. Pretreatment with genistein for 48 h prior to radiation enhanced G2/M phase arrest of the cell cycle only in ME180 cells, but not in CaSki cells. Such increased radiosensitivity correlated with inhibition of Mcl-1 expression and suppression of activated pAkt levels. However, another bioactive soy isoflavone daidzein had no effect of radiosensitivity in either CaSki or ME180 cells [35] (Table 2). Much higher doses of genistein (200 μM) led to augmentation of radiation-induced inhibition of viability of CaSki cells, with increase in G2/M phase arrest of cell cycle progression and elevated levels of p53 and p21. In addition, combined treatment resulted in more apoptotic death than either single modality alone, described by upregulation of Bax and downregulation of Bcl-2 proteins, release of cytochrome c from mitochondria to the cytosol and activation of caspases-8 and -3. This was mediated by stimulation of radiation-induced ROS production by genistein. Increase in cyclooxygenase-2 (COX-2) expression and concomitant generation of prostaglandin E2 (PGE2) followed to irradiation of cells were almost completely prevented by pretreatment with genistein. Moreover, cotreatment suppressed the transcripts of E6 and E7 levels, probably allowing restoration of p53 and p21^{WAF1} functions [66]. Pretreatment with genistein enhanced radiosensitivity also in another high-risk HPV-infected human cervical cancer cell line, HeLa (HPV18-positive). The antiproliferative rate of cells treated with combination of genistein and radiation was significantly higher compared to those cells that were treated with either modality alone. Genistein treatment in conjunction with radiation led to significantly increased arrest of cells in the G2/M phase and subsequent apoptotic death, with suppression of radiation-induced survivin expression [36]. Thus, although *in vivo* preclinical studies are urgently needed to confirm the *in vitro* findings about radiosensitizing potential of genistein in cervical cancer models, current data provide promise that combined use of genistein and radiotherapy might improve the response of patients to the treatment and thereby enhance therapeutic outcome.

4.1.1.6. Esophageal Cancer

Esophageal cancer is one of the most common tumor types of the gastrointestinal tract, with an estimated 572 034 new cases in 2018 in the whole world [1]. The most common type of esophageal cancer is esophageal squamous cell carcinoma accounting for about 90% of all esophageal cancer cases, with esophageal adenocarcinoma being another common histological tumor type [31, 32]. Esophageal cancer is usually treated by surgery, radiotherapy, chemotherapy and combination of these modalities [31].

Incubation with genistein (30 µM) greatly enhanced radiosensitivity in two human esophageal squamous cell cancer cell lines, TE-1 with mutant p53 and TE-2 with wild-type p53. This radiosensitizing activity of genistein was mediated by blocking radiation-induced activation of survival signals, i.e., p42/p44 ERK and Akt pathways, accompanied by decrease in cyclin D1 level. Combined treatment of TE-2 cells (but still not TE-1 cells) with genistein and radiation led to a significant increase in apoptotic death, characterized by enhanced Bax and reduced Bcl-2 levels and cleavage of PARP protein. Thus, the mode of cell death in p53 wild-type and p53 mutant esophageal squamous cell carcinoma cells was still somewhat different [69] (Table 2). Nevertheless, these data indicate that genistein could be an important complementary therapeutic agent for enhancing radiation effect in esophageal cancer treatment.

4.1.1.7. Colorectal Cancer

Colorectal cancer is the third leading cause of cancer incidence in the world, with an estimated 1 800 977 new cases in 2018 [1]. Risk of colorectal cancer is continuously increasing due to admission of Western lifestyle featured by changes in dietary habits and reduced physical activity [37].

Genistein used in conjunction with ionizing radiation produced an antagonistic or slightly additive antiproliferative effects in HCT116 human colorectal cancer cells. Pretreatment with genistein for 24 h only weakly suppressed EGFR activity upregulated by radiotherapy, and enhanced radiation-induced activation of Akt and ERK1/2 survival signaling pathways [68] (Table 2). These somewhat unexpectant findings argue against genistein supplementation of colorectal cancer patients undergoing radiotherapeutic treatment.

4.1.1.8. Hepatocellular Carcinoma

Hepatocellular carcinoma is one of the most frequent malignancies worldwide, with an estimated 841 080 new cases in 2018 [1]. The incidence of this tumor type is highest in developing countries of East Asia [8, 51].

In combination with radiation, genistein caused an increase in radiation-induced cell death in Reuber H35 rat hepatoma cells, associated with decreased repair of DNA damage. At that, incubation of cells with genistein until 24 h after irradiation was critical to achieve enhancement of radiation-caused cell killing [84] (Table 2). Further studies combining genistein with ionizing radiation in human hepatocellular carcinoma cell lines are highly needed.

4.1.1.9. Sarcoma

Although sarcoma is a very rare tumor, this disease is especially complex due to high biological and molecular heterogeneity. The prognosis of sarcoma patients has still remained poor [61].

Pretreatment with genistein (10 µM) was shown to augment the response of murine S180 soft tissue sarcoma cells to ionizing radiation. Radiation treatment combined with genistein suppressed the activity of DNA-PKs resulting in disturbances of homologous recombination and non-homologous end-joining DNA repair mechanisms, eventually leading to decrease in cell survival and increase in apoptotic death.

Induction of apoptosis was accompanied by upregulation of Bax, downregulation of Bcl-2 and release of cytochrome c from mitochondria into the cytoplasm. In addition, combined treatment of S180 tumor-bearing mice with genistein and radiation led to considerably smaller tumors with higher apoptotic rates and reduced blood vessels compared to counterparts treated with radiation alone [61] (Table 2). Further studies should determine whether the radiosensitizing effect of genistein observed in murine sarcoma preclinical models is valid also in human soft tissue sarcoma cells.

4.1.1.10. Glioblastoma Multiforme

Glioblastoma multiforme is the most common type of primary brain tumors in adults. Despite aggressive treatment modalities, including surgery, radiotherapy and chemotherapy, the prognosis of patients suffering from this highly invasive malignancy is still unfavorable and complete removal of tumors is mostly impossible. Increased resistance to conventional therapies also contributes to poor prognosis [77, 85].

Effect of genistein on response of U87MG human glioblastoma multiforme cells to ionizing radiation was shown to be substantially dependent on genistein concentration. In fact, genistein at 10 μM in combination with irradiation (either single dose or fractionated) enhanced survival fraction of malignant cells and behaved as a radioprotector. In contrast, pretreatment of cells with 50 μM genistein for 30 h before irradiation led to a greater decrease in cell proliferation and survival compared to either single modality, thereby acting as a potential radiosensitizer [77] (Table 2). As 10 μM plasma concentrations can be achieved by administration of genistein-rich dietary supplements, and considering also the capability of genistein to rapidly pass through the blood brain barrier [77], glioblastoma patients undergoing radiotherapy should be cautious when consuming genistein supplements (at least in its pure form).

4.1.1.11. Chronic Myelogenous Leukemia

Chronic myelogenous leukemia is a myeloproliferative disorder characterized by the clonal expansion of pluripotent hematopoietic stem cells [52].

Genistein at higher doses (50 µM) enhanced radiation-induced apoptosis in K562 human chronic myelogenous leukemia cells by promoting arrest in cell cycle progression [86] (Table 2). However, lower doses of genistein (25 µM) contrarily decreased the radiosensitivity and protected K562 cells from radiation-induced cell death leading to increased cell survival. This radioprotecting effect was achieved through a prolonged maintenance of G2 phase arrest and inhibition of caspase-3 activity by genistein [52, 87]. The ability of genistein to enhance the expression and enzymatic activity of thymidine kinase 1 (TK1) could essentially contribute to modulation of radiation-induced toxicity in K562 cells [52]. Based on these findings, genistein supplements (at least in its isolated purified form) can enhance the radioresistance of chronic myelogenous leukemia cells and thereby result in reduced therapeutic outcome.

Altogether, several *in vitro* and *in vivo* preclinical studies have suggested a potential of combining genistein (or soy isoflavones formulations) with radiation therapy for the treatment of various human tumor types, including localized prostate carcinoma, renal cell carcinoma, non-small cell lung cancer, breast cancer, cervical cancer and esophageal squamous cell carcinoma. Such radiosensitizing effect of genistein represents a rather unique phenomenon, being independent on the presence of androgen receptors in prostate cancer cells, estrogen receptors in breast cancer cells, or KRAS and EGFR mutation status in non-small cell lung cancer cells. Therefore, design of clinical trials is important to improve the therapeutic outcome of radiation treatment of cancer patients in the future. However, there are still some adverse effects published about combining genistein and irradiation, arguing against the use of this soy isoflavone (at least in its pure form) by patients suffering from colorectal cancer, glioblastoma and myeloid leukemia before receiving radiotherapy. Whether this undesired radioprotecting action observed with pure genistein will be recapitulated also with natural soy isoflavones formulations, which are actually used in human interventions, remains to be clarified.

4.1.2. Equol

Equol is the major metabolite of soy isoflavone daidzein and is produced by the gut microflora (Table 1). Production of equol essentially depends on the presence of specific intestinal bacteria, whereas only about one-third to half of all adult individuals are able to convert daidzein to equol. It has been suggested that equol can give an important contribution to anticancer properties of soy [75].

4.1.2.1. Breast Cancer

Pretreatment with equol (50 µM) was shown to sensitize both ERα-negative MDA-MB-231 human breast cancer cells as well as ERα-positive T47D human breast cancer cells to ionizing radiation. Combined treatment with equol and radiation promoted radiation-induced DNA damage and apoptotic death, thereby reducing the surviving fraction of irradiated cells. The radiosensitizing potential of equol was stronger in MDA-MB-231 cells that are high-grade, invasive and more resistant to radiation treatment alone as compared to poorly or noninvasive T47D cells [75], suggesting that equol can confer enhancement of radiotherapeutic efficacy of breast tumors sensitizing radioresistant clones (Table 2).

4.1.3. Biochanin A

Biochanin A is a methylated genistein derivative that can be found in large amounts in red clover [44] (Table 1).

4.1.3.1. Colon Cancer
Colon cancer is a common malignancy with continuously growing global incidence rate associated with changes in the human diet. In 2018, there was an estimated 1 096 601 new colon cancer cases all over the world [1].

Combined treatment of HT29 human colon cancer cells with biochanin A and radiation led to a significant decrease in cell proliferation, accompanied by increase in intracellular ROS production, lipid peroxidation and apoptotic death. Mitochondrial membrane potential and caspase-3 activity were remarkably enhanced after combined treatment compared to either single modality. Biochanin A acted as a typical prooxidant in colon cancer cells when combined with radiation, yielding a substantial enhancement of radiotoxicity [44] (Table 2). Regarding to continuous increase in colon cancer cases worldwide, further studies of radiosensitizing potential of biochanin A on colon cancer preclinical models are imperative.

4.1.4. Alpinumisoflavone

Alpinumisoflavone is one of the major bioactive components of a traditional Chinese medicinal herb *Derris eriocarpa* F. C. How [31] (Table 1).

4.1.4.1. Esophageal Cancer
Pretreatment with alpinumisoflavone (5 µM) could significantly enhance the radiosensitivity in human esophageal squamous cell

carcinoma cell lines, KYSE30 and Eca109. Combined treatment with alpinumisoflavone and radiation led to a greater DNA damage, G2/M phase cell cycle blockade and apoptosis compared to either modality alone. This effect was achieved through aggravation of ROS production and oxidative stress, regulated by marked suppression of radiation-induced increase in Nrf2 nuclear expression and downstream antioxidant enzymes by alpinumisoflavone. In addition, alpinumisoflavone augmented radiation-induced inhibition of tumor growth also in Eca109 xenograft-bearing nude mice, revealing significantly smaller tumors [31] (Table 2). Thus, alpinumisoflavone can function as a potent radiosensitizer for human esophageal squamous cell carcinoma, augmenting the ability of radiation to harm malignant cells and holding therapeutic potential for possible clinical use in the future.

4.2. FLAVANOLS

4.2.1. Epigallocatechin 3-Gallate

Epigallocatechin 3-gallate (EGCG) is the most abundant polyphenol in green tea [76] (Table 1). Chemopreventive and anticancer properties of EGCG have been, at least partially, related to its antioxidant and free radical scavenging abilities [76]. EGCG is one of the most frequently consumed dietary supplements by cancer patients, but still only a few studies have evaluated the potential modulation of radiotherapeutic efficacy by EGCG [7, 70, 88].

The plasma concentrations of EGCG are generally less than 1 µM after regular intake of green tea [76]. Somewhat higher levels can be attained following consumption of EGCG supplements, such as Polyphenon E [67]. For instance, the average maximum plasma levels of EGCG reached 7.4 µM after oral administration of EGCG to humans [67]. Essentially higher levels of EGCG have been measured in the oral cavity after drinking green tea, with salivary EGCG levels ranging from 10.5 µM to 48 µM. Moreover, holding highly concentrated green tea extract for a while in the oral cavity led to salivary EGCG concentrations even up to 370 µM [89].

4.2.1.1. Breast Cancer

Treatment of MDA-MB-231 human breast cancer cells with EGCG (5 µM, 10 µM) revealed a significant potentiation of radiation-induced decrease in cell viability, accompanied by suppression of NF-κB level and Akt activation [67] (Table 3). Furthermore, oral administration of 400 mg EGCG three times daily to breast cancer patients undergoing radiation treatment led to changes in several blood parameters. Serum levels of vascular endothelial growth factor (VEGF) and hepatocyte growth factor (HGF) were significantly decreased, and activities of matrix metalloproteinases (MMPs)-2 and -9 were reduced in patients who received EGCG supplements under radiotherapy compared to radiation-only treated counterparts. As elevated levels of these parameters are closely related to the progression, invasion and metastasis of breast cancer, their reduction suggests an improved clinical prognosis [67]. These data exhibit the potential of green tea polyphenol EGCG to be an important therapeutic adjuvant for treatment of breast cancer, augmenting radiotherapeutic efficacy and restricting tumor progression and spread. However, using Mca-IV murine breast carcinoma bearing mice model, no significant radiomodulating effects of EGCG were observed [7].

4.2.1.2. Cervical Cancer

Pretreatment with high concentrations of EGCG (100 µM, 200 µM) potentiated the response of HeLa human cervical cancer cells to ionizing radiation, leading to a significant decrease in proliferation and increase in apoptotic death compared to treatment with either modality alone [64] (Table 3). Further studies are needed to ascertain whether the radiosensitizing effect of EGCG could be dependent on the HPV subtype integrated into human cervical cancer cells and to further evaluate the therapeutic potential of EGCG as possible adjuvant agent for radiation treatment of cervical tumors.

4.2.1.3. Prostate Cancer

Physiologically achievable doses of EGCG (1.5-7.5 µM) significantly inhibited ionizing radiation-induced apoptosis in DU145 human prostate cancer cells, thereby acting as a radioprotector. The inhibitory effect on radiotherapeutic efficacy was strongest when EGCG was added 30 minutes before radiation. Combined treatment with EGCG and radiation induced enhanced levels of manganese superoxide dismutase (MnSOD) which could neutralize ROS produced by radiotherapy, attenuate radiotoxicity and confer radioresistance [76] (Table 3). Thus, pre-exposure to EGCG could prevent radiation-induced death of prostate cancer cells due to direct antioxidant effects of EGCG, suggesting that nutrient antioxidants can adversely affect cancer treatment, and warning prostate cancer patients against intake of supplements rich in EGCG when undergoing radiotherapy. Further studies should determine whether 1) this radioprotecting action of EGCG is dependent on the presence of androgen receptors in prostate cancer cells, 2) the undesired radioprotecting effects of EGCG are reproduced with green tea extracts containing besides EGCG also other structurally different flavanols, and 3) the adverse action of EGCG is recapitulated in prostate tumor models *in vivo*. If so, then prostate cancer patients should be warned against abundant drinking of green tea when receiving radiotherapy.

Table 3. Effects of flavanols on cancer radiotherapeutic efficacy

Agent	Cancer site	Biological system	Method	Assay conditions		Effect	Ref.
Epicatechin, EC	Brain	U87 human glioblastoma-astrocytoma cells	Colony formation	Pretreatment with EC (20 µM) for 1h, irradiation (2-8 Gy), incubation for 24h before assay	↑	Increase in radiosensitivity, decrease in surviving fraction	[18]
	Pancreas	MIA PaCa-2 human pancreatic epithelial carcinoma cells	Colony formation	Pretreatment with EC (20 µM) for 1h, irradiation (2-8 Gy), incubation for 24h before assay	↑	Increase in radiosensitivity, decrease in surviving fraction	[18]
		Panc-1 human pancreatic epithelial carcinoma cells		Pretreatment with EC (20 µM) for 1h, irradiation (2-8 Gy), incubation for 24h before assay	↑	Decrease in surviving fraction. Increase in cleaved caspase-3; stimulation of Chk2 phosphorylation and p21 expression	[18]
Epigallo-catechin 3-gallate, EGCG	Blood	K562 human chronic myelogenous leukemia cells	Counting	Pretreatment with EGCG (25-200 µM) for 1h before X-ray irradiation (2, 4, 6 Gy)	↑	Inhibition of proliferation, increase in apoptosis	[64]
		IM-9 human multiple myeloma cells		Pretreatment with EGCG (10-200 µM) for 1h before X-ray irradiation (2, 4, 6 Gy)	↑	Inhibition of proliferation, increase in apoptosis	[64]
		EOL-1 human eosinophilic leukemia cells		Treatment with EGCG (25 µM) and X-ray irradiation (4 Gy)	↑	Decrease in proliferation, increase in apoptosis	[63]
	Brain	U87 human glioblastoma cells	Counting	Pretreatment with EGCG (25 µM) for 6h before photon irradiation (10 Gy)	↑	Inhibition of proliferation. Downregulation of radiation-induced RhoA, reversal of cytoprotective effect of survivin	[42]

Table 3. (Continued)

Agent	Cancer site	Biological system	Method	Assay conditions	Effect		Ref.
	Breast	MDA-MB-231 human breast cancer cells (highly metastatic)	Counting	Treatment with EGCG (5, 10 µM) plus γ-irradiation (8 Gy) for 36h	↑	Reduction of cell viability. Decrease in NF-κB level and AKT phosphorylation	[67]
		Implantation of stage IV murine cancer (Mca-IV) cells into right hindleg of female CH3 mice	Tumor growth analysis	Feeding of mice with EGCG (658 µg/g bw) containing diet for 30 days, implantation of tumor, irradiation (60-85 Gy) after 10-15 days	~	No radiomodifying effect on tumor control	[7]
		Patients with locally advanced (T3, T4, and/or N0-N3) non-inflammatory breast cancer undergoing radiotherapy		Oral administration of EGCG (400 mg, 3 times daily) during 5 weeks radiotherapy cycles and 3 weeks post-radiotherapy cycle	↑	Decrease in serum levels of VEGF, HGF and MMPs-9/-2 activity	[67]
	Cervix	HeLa human cervical carcinoma cells	Counting	Pretreatment with EGCG (100, 200 µM) for 1h before X-ray irradiation (2, 4, 6 Gy)	↑	Inhibition of proliferation, increase in apoptosis	[64]
	Colorectum	HCT116 human colorectal cancer cells	CCK-8, colony formation	Pretreatment with EGCG (12.5 µM) for 24h before X-ray irradiation (2 Gy) (colony assay); incubation with EGCG with simultaneous exposure to irradiation (CCK-8)	↑	Inhibition of growth and colony number. Increase in Nrf2 nuclear translocation, LC3 and caspase-9 levels	[56]
	Mouth	OSC-2 human oral squamous cell carcinoma cells	MTT	Pretreatment with EGCG (12.5, 25, 50 µM) for 24h before γ-irradiation (5, 10 Gy)	→	Increase in viability. Reversal of radiation-induced inhibition of DNA synthesis	[89]
	Prostate	DU145 human prostate cancer cells (androgen non-responsive)	Counting	Pretreatment with EGCG (1.5-7.5 µM) for 0.5h before irradiation (3.5 Gy) for 3 consecutive days	→	Decrease in radiation-induced apoptosis. Increase in MnSOD levels	[76]

4.2.1.4. Oral Cancer

Oral squamous cell carcinoma is the most frequent malignancy affecting the oral cavity. The poor prognosis of this disease has been associated with a common resistance of oral squamous cell carcinoma cells to therapeutic modalities used in clinical settings, including radiotherapy [34].

Pretreatment of OSC-2 human oral squamous cell carcinoma cells with physiologically attainable salivary doses of EGCG (12.5-50 µM) for 24 h followed by irradiation led to protection against radiotoxicity. EGCG when combined with radiation completely reversed radiation-induced inhibition of DNA synthesis and significantly increased cellular viability [89] (Table 3). Thus, administration of EGCG prior to or during oral cancer radiotherapy might lead to protection of tumoral cells by accelerating cellular proliferation. If these findings will be reproduced with green tea extracts containing several other flavanols in addition to EGCG, it would be reasonable to recommend oral cancer patients to avoid regular drinking of green tea when undergoing radiotherapy. It is clear that the combination of EGCG/green tea intake and oral cancer therapy requires further in detail evaluation.

4.2.1.5. Colorectal Cancer

EGCG augmented the sensitivity of HCT116 human colorectal cancer cells to radiation treatment. Combination of EGCG (12.5 µM) and radiation resulted in a significant inhibition of cellular growth and survival compared to either treatment alone. This radiosensitizing effect was achieved through increasing nuclear translocation of Nrf2, and induction of LC3 (autophagic marker) and caspase-9 expression (apoptotic marker) [56] (Table 3).

4.2.1.6. Glioblastoma

Pretreatment with EGCG (25 µM) potentiated radiation-induced decrease in proliferation of U87 human glioblastoma cells by targeting prosurvival intracellular pathways. In fact, EGCG led to suppression of radiation-induced increase in survivin and RhoA protein expression, thus reversing cytoprotective effect of survivin towards ionizing radiation [42] (Table 3). Moreover, EGCG could sensitize also brain tumor-derived endothelial cells to irradiation treatment, demonstrated by enhanced inhibition of human brain microvascular endothelial cells survival after combined treatment with EGCG and irradiation through augmentation of necrotic death [40]. Considering the knowledge that EGCG can cross the blood brain barrier and rapidly get to the brain [63], these findings provide some promise that EGCG could be used as an adjuvant agent for radiotherapeutic treatment of radioresistant and highly vascularized high-grade gliomas, enhancing the proportion of cells in radiosensitive state.

4.2.1.7. Blood Cancer

Combined treatment with EGCG and ionizing radiation resulted in a significant decrease in proliferation and increase in apoptosis in K562 human chronic myelogenous leukemia cells, EOL-1 human eosinophilic leukemia cells and IM-9 human multiple myeloma cells as compared to the treatments by either modality alone [63, 64] (Table 3). At that, EGCG either alone or in conjunction with a low dose of irradiation could almost completely prevent the growth of IM-9 cells [64]. Thus, EGCG can cause augmentation of radiation toxicity in diverse blood cancer cells to a different degree depending on the origin of cells, highlighting the need for further preclinical studies.

Altogether, action of EGCG on radiotherapeutic efficacy seems to largely depend on the cancer type, cell line and EGCG concentrations. Whereas *in vitro* preclinical studies have suggested radiosensitizing effects of EGCG in human breast, cervical and colorectal cancer, glioblastoma, multiple myeloma, myeloid and eosinophilic leukemia cells, this abundant green tea polyphenol might behave as a radioprotector in prostate and oral cancer cells, possibly attenuating therapeutic efficacy and promoting disease progression.

4.2.2. Epicatechin

Epicatechin is a natural flavanol present in many fruits and vegetables, especially in cocoa and green tea [18] (Table 1).

4.2.2.1. Pancreatic Cancer

Pancreatic cancer is one of the most lethal cancer types today with a mortality rate almost equal to its incidence. Indeed, in 2018, there were an estimated 458 918 new pancreatic cancer cases with 432 242 deaths worldwide [1].

Pretreatment with epicatechin enhanced radiotherapeutic efficacy in human pancreatic cancer cell lines Panc-1 and MIA Paca-2, reducing surviving fraction of cells after irradiation. Combined treatment of Panc-1 cells with epicatechin and radiation resulted in an enhanced p21 expression, checkpoint kinase 2 (Chk2) phosphorylation and caspase-3 cleavage as compared to radiation-only treated cells, suggesting that radiosensitizing action of epicatechin was achieved by intervening in DNA damage response, cell cycle progression and apoptotic death [18] (Table 3). Considering the high lethality of pancreatic tumors, possibilities to include epicatechin as a promising adjuvant agent for pancreatic cancer treatment in combination with radiotherapy should be further evaluated.

4.2.2.2. Glioblastoma

Epicatechin sensitized U87 human glioblastoma cells toward ionizing radiation with a significant enhancement of radiation-induced cell death. Meanwhile, epicatechin did not enhance radiotoxicity in human normal fibroblasts, showing that the radiosensitizing effect of epicatechin was specific to malignant cells [18] (Table 3). Taking into account that both EGCG and epicatechin behaved as potential radiosensitizers for human glioblastoma cells and presuming that these two flavanols could enhance radiotherapeutic efficacy by affecting different intracellular pathways, synergistic effects could be expected when combining radiation with green tea extracts. Epicatechin, EGCG and possibly also green tea extracts are promising candidates to improve therapeutic outcome of glioma patients by potentiating conventional radiotherapy.

4.3. Flavonols

4.3.1. Quercetin

Quercetin is a ubiquitous natural flavonoid found in various fruits, vegetables, nuts and grains, such as apples, berries, onions and tomatoes [15, 41, 85] (Table 1). Quercetin can exert several anticancer activities through affecting multiple cellular pathways [3, 85].

Plasma levels of quercetin remain at nanomolar range (usually less than 100 nM) after common dietary intake; however, micromolar doses could be achieved following consumption of supplements rich in quercetin [41]. Besides being cheap and readily available, quercetin has been considered to be completely safe for humans at doses up to 1 g/day, making it an attractive agent for preclinical studies, both alone as well as in combination with conventional anticancer modalities [41, 85].

4.3.1.1. Brain Cancer
The addition of quercetin (25 μM) to irradiation resulted in a greater reduction of cell survival and activation of apoptosis in two human glioblastoma cell lines, U251 and DBTRG-05, as compared to the treatment with either single modality. Induction of apoptosis was

characterized by increased cleavage of caspase-3 and PARP proteins, regulated through a significant decrease in Akt activation [85] (Table 4). These findings might be especially important, considering the ability of quercetin to effectively cross the blood brain barrier and accumulate in the brain [41]. Furthermore, quercetin at low micromolar doses achievable by oral intake (1 µM) was shown to radiosensitize also different human medulloblastoma cell lines, DAOY, D283-Med and D458-Med, leading to a significant decrease in cell growth after combined treatment with quercetin and radiation. This action of quercetin was specific for malignant cells, as no sensitizing effects were detected in normal human fibroblasts or neuronal precursor cells. In addition, administration of quercetin in combination with irradiation significantly improved radiotherapeutic efficacy *in vivo* and prolonged survival of D283-Med orthotopic tumor bearing mice, suggesting that quercetin might be a putative radiosensitizer for medulloblastoma as the most common pediatric brain malignancy. The lack of detecting radiosensitizing effect of quercetin in two primary medulloblastoma cell cultures, VU371 and ICb-1299MB, was probably associated with the high cellular radiosensitivity, letting no actual window for action of quercetin in experimental conditions [41]. Thus, the addition of quercetin to radiation treatment might provide novel benefits for patients suffering from glioblastoma or medulloblastoma to improve the clinical outcome and prolong survival. Clinical trials are needed to further evaluate the use of quercetin as an adjuvant agent for radiotherapeutic treatment of brain tumors.

4.3.1.2. Breast Cancer

Pretreatment with quercetin (10 µM) enhanced the response of MCF-7 human breast cancer cells to ionizing radiation. This radiosensitizing action of quercetin was mechanistically mediated via inhibition of ATM pathway that was activated in response to radiation-induced DNA damage, thereby prolonging the DNA repair processes and leading to decrease in cell survival [15] (Table 4). Further studies should evaluate whether this radiosensitizing effect of quercetin is common for breast tumors or could be dependent on the presence of estrogen receptors on malignant cells.

4.3.1.3. Ovarian Cancer

Ovarian cancer is one of the most common tumor types in women, with an estimated 295 414 new cases in 2018 worldwide [1].

Pre-exposure to high doses of quercetin (100 µM) potentiated radiation-induced cell death in two human ovarian cancer lines, A2780 and OV2008. Combined treatment with quercetin and radiation led to a prolonged DNA repair and increased number of DNA double stranded beaks, regulated by affecting the ATM signaling pathways. Augmentation of apoptotic death was further described by elevated levels of Bax, p53 and p21, and decrease in Bcl-2 expression. In OV2008 tumor xenograft model in nude mice, combined treatment with quercetin and radiation led to a greater suppression of tumor growth accompanied by an increase in p53 level and the number of γ-H2AX foci as compared to the treatment with ionizing radiation alone [3] (Table 4).

4.3.1.4. Cervical Cancer

Quercetin (10 µM) was shown to significantly augment the radiation-induced decrease in clonogenic survival of HeLa human cervical cancer cells. Mechanisms behind this radioenhancing effect involved abrogation of radiation-induced activation of ATM and ATM-mediated signaling, thereby suppressing DNA repair and resulting in enhancement of radiation-induced DNA double-strand breaks [15] (Table 4). Based on the current knowledge, it is still unclear whether the radiosensitizing action of quercetin is specific for high-risk HPV18 expressing HeLa cells or occurs also in other cervical cancer cells infected with different HPV subtypes.

4.3.1.5. Colorectal Cancer

Combined treatment of DLD1 human colorectal cancer cells with quercetin (10 µM) and radiation led to a greater decrease in cell survival as the treatment with either modality alone. Such increase in radiosensitivity was achieved through inhibition of ATM signaling and prolongation of DNA repair after exposure to quercetin, causing an extended retention of γ-H2AX foci. In addition, a significant increase in tumor growth delay was observed in irradiated DLD-1 xenografts bearing nude mice when intraperitoneally pretreated with quercetin [15] (Table 4). Thus, quercetin could enhance colorectal tumor radiosensitivity both *in vitro* and *in vivo* models, revealing the need for further clinical trials.

4.3.1.6. Hepatocellular Carcinoma

Quercetin caused an augmentation of radiation-induced death in Reuber H35 rat hepatoma cells. However, the enhancement of radiotoxicity was appeared only when quercetin was applied for until 24 h following radiation treatment [58, 84] (Table 4).

Altogether, quercetin can function as a potent radiosensitizer for different human solid tumor types, such as breast, ovarian, cervical and colorectal cancers as well as different brain tumors, demonstrated *in vitro* and *in vivo* preclinical assays. These findings clearly highlight the necessity for further clinical trials before possible use of this polyphenolic phytochemical as an adjuvant agent in clinical settings to improve the radiotherapeutic outcome of cancer patients.

4.3.2. Fisetin

Fisetin as a dietary flavonol with acceptable biosafety can be found in a wide range of fruits and vegetables [37] (Table 1). Fisetin is known by its diverse biological activities described in different tumoral cells [38].

Table 4. Effects of flavonols on cancer radiotherapeutic efficacy

Agent	Cancer site	Biological system	Method	Assay conditions	Effect	Ref.
Fisetin, FIS	Colon	s.c. injection of murine colon cancer CT-26 cells in the hind legs of male BALB/c nude mice	Tumor growth analysis	Intratumoral injection of FIS (5 mg/kg) on days 0 and 7; irradiation of tumors on days 2-6 (2 Gy/day)	↑ Suppression of tumor growth	[37]
	Colorectum	HT-29 human colorectal cancer cells	Counting, colony formation	Pretreatment with FIS (25, 50 μM) for 24h before X-ray irradiation (2, 4, 6 Gy)	↑ Reduction of survival fraction and proliferation. Prolongation and increase in radiation-induced G2/M arrest. Suppression of radiation-induced γ-H2AX phosphorylation and Chk2 activation. Increase in apoptosis (activation of caspase-3, PARP cleavage). Increase in radiation-induced p38 MAPK, decrease in pAKT and pERK1/2	[38]
		s.c. injection of human colorectal cancer HCT116 cells in the hind legs of male BALB/c nude mice	Tumor growth analysis	Intratumoral injection of FIS (5 mg/kg) on days 0 and 7; irradiation of tumors on days 2-6 (2 Gy/day)	↑ Complete inhibition of tumor growth, probably through downregulation of securin (no increase in radiation efficacy in securin-null cell-formed xenograft tumors)	[37]
Icariin, ICA	Colorectum	HT29 human colorectal cancer cells	Colony formation	Pretreatment with ICA (25 μM) for 4h before X-ray irradiation (6, 10 Gy) for 3h	↑ Reduction of survival. Increase in G2/M arrest and apoptosis. Inhibition of radiation-induced NF-κB activation and expression of downstream genes (IAP, Bcl-xL, Bcl-2, cyclin D1)	[47]
		HCT116 human colorectal cancer cells		Pretreatment with ICA (25 μM) for 4h before X-ray irradiation (6, 10 Gy) for 3h	↑ Reduction of survival. Increase in G2/M arrest and apoptosis. Inhibition of radiation-induced NF-κB activation and expression of downstream genes (IAP, Bcl-xL, Bcl-2, cyclin D1)	[47]

Agent	Cancer site	Biological system	Method	Assay conditions	Effect		Ref.
		Inoculation of HCT116 cells into the thigh of right hind leg of athymic BALB/c (nu/mu) mice	Tumor growth analysis	Daily oral administration of ICA (40 mg/kg); irradiation (4 Gy) given 1h after ICA twice weekly for 3 weeks	↑	Regression of tumor, decrease in tumor volume	[47]
Icaritin, ICT	Breast	4T1 murine breast cancer cells	Colony formation	Treatment with ICT (3, 6 μM) and irradiation (6, 8 Gy)	↑	Synergistic suppression of reproductive growth. Increase in G2/M arrest and apoptosis. Inhibition of radiation-induced ERK1/2 and AKT activation	[17]
Kaempferol, KAE	Lung	A549 human lung carcinoma cells	MTT, colony formation	Pretreatment with KAE (14 μM in MTT, 56 μM in colony assay) for 48h before photon irradiation (2-12 Gy)	↑	Decrease in cell growth and clonogenic survival. Inhibition of PI3K and ERK phosphorylation	[5]
		s.c. injection of A549 cells in BALB/c nude mice near the left hind leg	Tumor growth analysis	Pretreatment with KAE (56 μM) for 4h before radiation (4 Gy)	↑	Suppression of tumor growth, decrease in tumor volume. Inhibition of AKT/PI3K and ERK pathways, increase in caspase-3 inducing apoptosis	[5]
Myricetin, MYR	Lung	H1299 human non-small cell lung cancer	Colony formation, CCK-8	Addition of MYR (25 μM) for 1h before X-ray irradiation (2-8 Gy)	↑	Decrease in surviving fraction and proliferation. Enhancement of apoptosis (increase in caspase-3)	[62]
		A549 human non-small cell lung cancer cells		Addition of MYR (25 μM) for 1h before X-ray irradiation (2-8 Gy)	↑	Decrease in surviving fraction and proliferation. Enhancement of apoptosis (increase in caspase-3)	[62]
		s.c. injection of A549 cells in the dorsal scapular region of female BALB/C nude mice	Tumor growth analysis	i.p. administration of MYR (20 mg/kg once daily for 12 days) 1h before fractionated irradiation (2 Gy for 10 times)	↑	Suppression of tumor growth speed, decrease in tumor volume	[62]

Table 4. (Continued)

Agent	Cancer site	Biological system	Method	Assay conditions	Effect		Ref.
Quercetin, QUE	Brain	DBTRG-05 human glioblastoma cells	Colony formation, MTT	Pretreatment with QUE (25 µM) for 1h before radiation (4 Gy), incubation for 48h (MTT) or 7 days (colony assay)	↑	Reduction of cell viability and clonogenic survival. Increase in apoptosis (increase in caspase-3 and cleaved PARP through decrease in Akt activation)	[85]
		U251 human glioblastoma cells		Pretreatment with QUE (25 µM) for 1h before radiation (4 Gy), incubation for 48h (MTT) or 7 days (colony assay)	↑	Reduction of cell viability and clonogenic survival. Increase in apoptosis (increase in caspase-3 and cleaved PARP through decrease in Akt activation)	[85]
		D283-Med human medulloblastoma cells	Counting, colony formation	Pretreatment with QUE (1 µM) for 0.5h before irradiation (1-4 Gy)	↑	Reduction of cell growth and clonogenic survival	[41]
		D458-Med human medulloblastoma cells		Pretreatment with QUE (1 µM) for 0.5h before irradiation (1-4 Gy)	↑	Reduction of clonogenic survival	[41]
		DAOY human medulloblastoma cells	Counting	Pretreatment with QUE (1 µM) for 0.5h before irradiation (4 Gy)	↑	Reduction of cell growth	[41]
		ICb-1299MB primary medulloblastoma cells	Cell Titer Glo	Pretreatment with QUE (1 µM) for 0.5h before irradiation (0.7 Gy)	~	No effect on radiation response	[41]
		VU371 human primary medulloblastoma cells		Pretreatment with QUE (1 µM) for 0.5h before irradiation (0.7 Gy)	~	No effect on radiation response	[41]

Agent	Cancer site	Biological system	Method	Assay conditions	Effect		Ref.
		Stereotactic injection of D283-Med cells into cerebellum of female athymic nude-Fox1nu mice	Tumor growth analysis	i.p. administration of QUE (100 mg/kg) at 30 min and 60 min before or after irradiation, 0h and 24h after irradiation (4 Gy)	Improvement of radiation efficacy. Extension of animal survival	↑	[41]
	Breast	MCF-7 human breast cancer cells	Colony formation	Pretreatment with QUE (10 µM) for 1h before X-ray irradiation (2, 4, 6 Gy); maintained for 24h	Decrease in colony survival. Inhibition of radiation-activated ATM-mediated signaling	↑	[15]
	Cervix	HeLa human cervix cancer cells	Colony formation	Pretreatment with QUE (10 µM) for 1h before X-ray irradiation (2, 4, 6 Gy); maintained for 24h	Decrease in colony survival. Prolonged presence of radiation-induced γ-H2AX and 53BP1 foci. Inhibition of radiation-activated ATM-mediated signaling	↑	[15]
	Colorectum	DLD1 human colorectal cancer cells	Colony formation	Pretreatment with QUE (10 µM) for 1h before X-ray irradiation (2, 4, 6 Gy); maintained for 24h	Decrease in colony survival. Prolonged presence of radiation-induced γ-H2AX foci. Inhibition of radiation-activated ATM-mediated signaling	↑	[15]
		s.c. injection of DLD1 tumor fragments in male athymic nu/nu mice	Tumor growth analysis	i.p. treatment with QUE (30 mg/kg/ day for 14 days), for 1h before irradiation (2 Gy/ fraction for 10 times)	Increase in tumor growth delay	↑	[15]
	Liver	Reuber H35 rat hepatoma cells	Colony formation	Addition of QUE (90 µM) for 0.5h before X-ray irradiation (2-8 Gy); continuing incubation for 23.5h	Reduction of cell survival	↑	[84]
		Reuber H35 rat hepatoma cells	Counting	Exposure to QUE after X-ray irradiation (0-6 Gy)	Increase in radiosensitivity	↑	[58]

Table 4. (Continued)

Agent	Cancer site	Biological system	Method	Assay conditions	Effect		Ref.
	Ovary	A2780 human ovarian cancer cells	Colony formation	Pretreatment with QUE (100 µM) for 24h before X-ray irradiation (2-10 Gy)	↑	Reduction of surviving fraction. Increase in apoptosis (increase in p53, p21, Bax; decrease in Bcl-2). Activation of ATM-mediated pathway	[3]
		OV2008 human ovarian cancer cells		Pretreatment with QUE (100 µM) for 24h before X-ray irradiation (2-10 Gy)	↑	Reduction of surviving fraction. Increase in DNA damage and apoptosis (increase in p53, p21, Bax; decrease in Bcl-2). Activation of ATM-mediated pathway	[3]
		s.c. injection of OV2008 cells in both right and left flanks of female athymic nude mice	Tumor growth analysis	Oral treatment with QUE (2 mg/day, once daily for 14 doses) for 1h before fractionated irradiation (2 Gy for 10 times)	↑	Inhibition of tumor growth. Increase in p53, CHOP and γ-H2AX levels	[3]
Rhamnetin, RHA	Lung	NCI-H460 human non-small cell lung cancer cells	Colony formation	Treatment with RHA (15 µM) and exposure to γ-irradiation (2 Gy)	↑	Suppression of proliferation. p53-dependent increase in miR-34a expression leading to downregulation of Notch-1, NF-κB and prosurvival proteins (cIAP1, cIAP2, survivin). Increase in apoptosis, reversal of radiation-induced EMT (increase in E-cadherin; decrease in vimentin, fibronectin)	[28]

Agent	Cancer site	Biological system	Method	Assay conditions	Effect		Ref.
		NCI-H1299 human non-small cell lung cancer cells	Colony formation	Treatment with RHA (15 µM) and exposure to γ-irradiation (2 Gy)	↑	Suppression of proliferation. p53-dependent increase in miR-34a expression leading to downregulation of Notch-1, NF-κB and prosurvival proteins (cIAP1, cIAP2, survivin). Increase in apoptosis, reversal of radiation-induced EMT (increase in E-cadherin; decrease in vimentin, fibronectin)	[28]
		Injection of NCI-H1299 cells in the flank of BALB/c athymic nude mice	Tumor growth analysis	i.p. administration of RHA (200 µg/kg bw daily for 25 days); irradiation (10 Gy, once a week for 3 times)	↑	Reduction of tumor volume. Increase in miR-34a, suppression of radiation-induced expression of Notch-1, prosurvival proteins (cIAP1, cIAP2, survivin) and EMT-related proteins (vimentin, fibronectin)	[28]
Rutin, RUT	Colon	HT-29 human colon adenocarcinoma cells		Pretreatment with RUT (80 µM) for 24h before X-ray irradiation (4 Gy)	↑	Increase in oxidative stress (TBARS), DNA damage and apoptosis (loss of mitochondrial membrane potential). Decrease in enzymatic antioxidants (SOD, CAT, GPx)	[49]
Syringetin, SYR	Lung	H1299 human non-small cell lung cancer cells	Colony formation	Pretreatment with SYR (20, 40 µM) for 3h before X-ray irradiation (9, 12 Gy); incubation for 21h before assay	↑	Reduction of survival fraction. Increase in apoptotic cells (activation of caspase-3)	[50]
		C3H/MCA clone 15 murine cancer cells		Pretreatment with SYR (20 µM) for 3h before X-ray irradiation (5, 8 Gy); incubation for 21h before assay	↑	Reduction of survival fraction	[50]

Table 4. (Continued)

Agent	Cancer site	Biological system	Method	Assay conditions	Effect	Ref.
Troxerutin, TRO	Prostate	DU145 human prostate cancer cells (radioresistant)	MTT	Pretreatment with TRO (0.5, 2, 5 mM) for 24h before γ-irradiation (4 Gy)	↑	Increase in radiation-induced cytotoxicity and apoptosis. Increase in ROS. Binding to minor groove of DNA, inducing DNA strand breaks	[27]
		PC-3 human prostate cancer cells (radiosensitive)		Pretreatment with TRO (0.5, 2, 5 mM) for 24h before γ-irradiation (4 Gy)	↑	Increase in radiation-induced cytotoxicity and apoptosis	[27]

4.3.2.1. Colorectal Cancer

Pretreatment with fisetin (25 μM, 50 μM) for 24 h significantly augmented radiation-induced decrease in proliferation and survival of HT-29 human colorectal cancer cells, which is a p53-mutant cell line. Exposure to fisetin in conjunction with radiation prolonged G2/M phase arrest of the cell cycle progression, suppressed DNA repair capability and enhanced radiation-induced apoptotic death characterized by elevated caspase-3 activation and PARP cleavage. Increase in radiation-induced p38 mitogen-activated protein kinase (MAPK) activation and decrease in the levels of activated Akt and ERK1/2 contributed to the potentiation of radiosensitivity by fisetin [38] (Table 4). Furthermore, intratumoral administration of fisetin in combination with radiation led to a complete inhibition of tumor growth in nude mice harboring HCT116 human colorectal cancer xenografts, probably via downregulation of oncoprotein securin as no radiosensitizing effects of fisetin appeared in securin-null HCT116 tumor bearing mice. Similarly, combined treatment of fisetin and radiation induced a greater suppression of tumor growth in mice implanted with CT-26 murine colon cancer cells as compared to the treatment with radiation alone [37]. These findings indicate that fisetin could be potentially developed as a novel radiosensitizer against human colorectal tumors. In the future, addition of fisetin as a safe adjuvant to radiotherapeutic treatment protocols might allow reduction of total radiation exposure of colorectal cancer patients conferring improvement of their quality of life.

4.3.3. Kaempferol

Kaempferol is a common natural flavonoid that is present in tea, vegetables and fruits, such as broccoli, Brussels sprouts, grapefruits and apples [5] (Table 1).

4.3.3.1. Non-Small Cell Lung Cancer

Pretreatment with kaempferol (14 μM, 56 μM) for 48 h before irradiation enhanced radiation-induced inhibition of cell growth and survival in A549 human non-small cell lung cancer cells. Potentiation of radiation-induced cell killing by kaempferol was achieved through suppression of the PI3K/Akt and ERK prosurvival pathways leading to activation of the mitochondrial apoptotic cascade. In addition, treatment of A549 tumor xenografts bearing nude mice with kaempferol for 4 h before radiation resulted in a significant inhibition of tumor growth and reduced tumor volume. Tumor sections treated with combination of kaempferol and radiation revealed morphological apoptotic changes accompanied by increase in caspase-3 expression, besides suppressed levels of activated PI3K, AKT and ERK proteins [5] (Table 4). Thus, kaempferol can function as a safe and potential radiosensitizer for treatment of non-small cell lung cancers, requiring further in detail evaluation.

4.3.4. Myricetin

Myricetin is a non-toxic dietary flavonoid present in a wide variety of fruits, vegetables, berries and medicinal herbs [62] (Table 1).

4.3.4.1. Non-Small Cell Lung Cancer

The application of myricetin (25 μM) for 1 h prior to radiation exposure enhanced radiosensitivity of human non-small cell lung cancer cells, A549 and H1299. Combined treatment with myricetin and radiation led to augmentation of radiation-induced suppression of cell proliferation and survival, and potentiated the apoptotic cell death with increased expression of caspase-3. *In vivo* results further demonstrated a significantly lowered tumor growth rate in irradiated A549 xenograft bearing mice when pretreated with myricetin as compared to radiation-only treated counterparts [62] (Table 4). These findings show that myricetin as a safe natural dietary compound can augment radiotherapeutic efficacy in treatment of human pulmonary tumors and point to the necessity of further studies.

4.3.5. Rhamnetin

Rhamnetin is a natural monomethylated derivative of quercetin (Table 1).

4.3.5.1. Non-Small Cell Lung Cancer

Rhamnetin (15 µM) was shown to potentiate radiation-induced suppression of cell proliferation in human non-small cell lung cancer cell lines, NCI-H460 and NCI-H1299. Treatment with rhamnetin downregulated radiation-induced Notch-1 overexpression, but not activation, via p53-dependent increase in tumor-suppressive microRNA, miR-34a. As a consequence, reduced Notch-1 expression led to downregulation of NF-κB prosurvival signaling pathways with significant decrease in the levels of apoptotic inhibitors (cIAP1, cIAP2, survivin), further promoting apoptotic cell death. In addition, miR-34a-mediated inhibition of Notch-1 expression by rhamnetin resulted also in suppression of radiation-induced epithelial-mesenchymal transition (EMT). Lung cancer cells treated with combination of rhamnetin and radiation revealed reduced migration by increasing the expression of epithelial marker E-cadherin and decreasing the levels of mesenchymal markers vimentin and fibronectin. Thus, rhamnetin prevented Notch-1-mediated radioresistance and EMT phenotypes in both NCI-H460 and NCI-H1299 cells. Moreover, radiosensitizing and EMT reversing effects of rhamnetin were confirmed also in *in vivo* conditions using NCI-H1299 xenograft mouse model. Combined treatment with rhamnetin and radiation resulted in a significant inhibition of tumor growth with reduced tumor volumes compared to the radiation treatment alone. Thereat, intraperitoneal administration of rhamnetin to irradiated tumor-bearing mice resulted in a significant reduction of radiation-induced expressions of Notch-1, antiapoptotic proteins and EMT-related proteins in the extracted tumor tissue lysates [28] (Table 4). Therefore, rhamnetin could be a promising radiosensitizer for enhancement of radiotherapeutic efficacy in the treatment of human non-small cell lung cancers, with Notch-1 as a novel important pharmacological target for further radiosensitizing studies.

4.3.6. Syringetin

Syringetin is a dimethylated derivative of myricetin, present in red grapes and red wine [50] (Table 1).

4.3.6.1. Non-Small Cell Lung Cancer

Syringetin (20 µM, 40 µM) augmented radiosensitivity in H1299 human non-small cell lung cancer cells and also C3H/MCA clone 15 murine cancer cells. Pre-exposure of H1299 cells to syringetin for 3 h before radiation led to an enhanced apoptotic death with increase in caspase-3 activation as compared to radiation treatment alone. This radiosensitizing effect of syringetin was independent on p53 status of H1299 cells, occurring both in wild-type p53- as well as mutant p53-transfected cells. Moreover, radioenhancing action of syringetin was more effective in malignant cells as compared to that of normal human lung fibroblast cells HFL-III [50] (Table 4). Therefore, syringetin as a safe natural compound could be useful for the development of novel efficient radiosensitizers to improve the therapeutic outcome of lung cancer patients.

4.3.7. Rutin

Rutin or quercetin 3-rutinoside is widely found in various plants, fruits and vegetables. The richest sources of rutin are buckwheat, citrus fruits and berries, including mulberries and cranberries [49] (Table 1).

4.3.7.1. Colon Cancer

Pretreatment with rutin (80 µM) augmented radiation-induced decrease in cell viability and increase in cell killing of HT-29 human colon cancer cells. Combined treatment with rutin and radiation led to an enhanced DNA damage and lipid peroxidation with elevated levels of thiobarbituric acid reactive substances (TBARS) as compared to the treatment with radiation alone. In addition, reduced antioxidant status was observed, as enzymatic activities of superoxide dismutase (SOD), catalase (CAT) and glutathione peroxidase (GPx) were suppressed leading to oxidative stress. As a result, apoptotic death cascade was triggered, characterized by alterations in nuclear morphology and a complete loss of mitochondrial membrane potential [49] (Table 4). Thus, rutin could boost radiation-induced oxidative stress in human colon adenocarcinoma cells and behave as a potent sensitizer for radiotherapy.

4.3.8. Troxerutin

Troxerutin or trihydroxyethylated rutin can be frequently found in the human diet, occurring in tea, coffee, cereal grains, and various fruits and vegetables [27] (Table 1).

4.3.8.1. Prostate Cancer

Pretreatment with high doses of troxerutin (0.5-5 mM) for 24 h enhanced radiation-induced cytotoxicity and apoptotic death in two human prostate cancer cell lines, DU145 and PC-3. In DU145 cells, combined treatment with troxerutin and radiation led to an increase in production of ROS and DNA damage as compared to either single modality. Thereat, troxerutin was able to bind to genomic DNA at minor groove, confer strand breaks and augment cancer cell killing in response to ionizing radiation [27] (Table 4). Thus, troxerutin has potential to be a potent adjuvant agent for prostate cancer radiotherapy.

4.3.9. Icaritin

Icaritin is a prenylated flavonol isolated from plants of the genus *Epimedium*, used in traditional Chinese medicine [17] (Table 1).

4.3.9.1. Breast Cancer

Icaritin (3 µM, 6 µM) in conjunction with radiation synergistically increased cell growth inhibition and killing of 4T1 murine breast cancer cells. Combined treatment of icaritin and radiation enhanced G2/M phase cell cycle arrest and augmented apoptotic death as compared to the treatment with radiation alone. This radiosensitizing effect of icaritin was achieved through suppression of radiation-induced activation of prosurvival molecules Akt and ERK1/2 to their basal levels, thereby disrupting the cellular protection processes against radiotoxicity [17] (Table 4). Further studies should elucidate whether the radiosensitizing effect of icaritin observed in highly aggressive murine breast cancer cells will be valid also for human breast tumors.

4.3.10. Icariin

Icariin is a prenylated flavonol glycoside, extracted from plants of the genus *Epimedium* [47] (Table 1). Icariin has been proven to be pharmacologically safe at its therapeutic doses [47].

4.3.10.1. Colorectal Cancer

Pre-exposure to icariin (25 µM) for 4 h enhanced radiation-induced antiproliferative effect and reduced clonogenic survival in two human colorectal cancer cell lines, HT29 and HCT116. Icariin in conjunction with radiation increased G2/M phase cell cycle arrest and promoted apoptotic death to a significantly greater extent than radiation treatment alone. This radioenhancing action of icariin was mediated through downregulation of radiation-induced activation NF-κB, and suppression of downstream antiapoptotic and pro-proliferative molecules, such as IAPs, Bcl-xL, Bcl-2 and cyclin D1. In addition, icariin was able to potentiate the radiotherapeutic efficacy also in HCT116 xenograft bearing mice, strengthening the radiation-induced tumor regression and resulting in significantly smaller malignant neoplasms [47] (Table 4). Thus, icariin could be a potent candidate for sensitizing colorectal tumors to radiotherapeutic treatment.

4.4. FLAVONES

4.4.1. Apigenin

Apigenin as one of the most common natural flavonoids is present in a variety of fruits and vegetables, especially in celery [54, 65] (Table 1).

4.4.1.1. Non-Small Cell Lung Cancer

Pretreatment with apigenin (40 µM) remarkably enhanced radiosensitivity in SQ5 human squamous cell carcinoma cells. The mechanism behind radioenhancing action of apigenin involved suppression of tumoral cell growth and potentiation of radiation-induced apoptosis, characterized by increase in WAF1/p21 level, decrease in Bcl-2 expression and cleavage of PARP protein [65] (Table 5). These findings indicate that apigenin might be useful for treatment of radioresistant lung tumors.

4.4.1.2. Laryngeal Cancer

Laryngeal carcinoma is a common type of head and neck tumors, with an estimated 177 422 new cases in 2018 worldwide [1]. Despite application of different treatment modalities, including surgical resection, radiotherapy and chemotherapy, the American Cancer Society has still reported a decrease in the 5-year survival rate of laryngeal cancer patients between 1975 and 2009 [54].

Apigenin was shown to improve the *in vivo* radiosensitivity of Hep-2 human laryngeal tumor bearing mice, reducing tumor size. This radiosensitizing effect was mediated through suppression of glucose transporter-1 (GLUT-1) expression by apigenin in irradiated tumor xenografts. GLUT-1 is a well-known hypoxic marker of various malignant neoplasms, whereas hypoxia can importantly contribute to the radioresistance phenotype of laryngeal carcinoma; the overexpression of GLUT-1 has been indeed previously reported to be associated with tumor radioresistance. Downregulation of GLUT-1 levels by apigenin were possibly regulated via suppression of the PI3K/Akt pathway [54] (Table 5). Thus, apigenin seems to be a promising radiosensitizer for management of human laryngeal carcinomas, suppressing the tendency of tumor cells to become radioresistant in response to hypoxic microenvironment.

4.4.1.3. Breast Cancer

Intraperitoneal administration of apigenin enhanced the *in vivo* radiosensitivity of murine Ehrlich carcinoma-bearing mice. Combined treatment with apigenin and radiation resulted in a synergistic suppression of tumor growth through downregulation of the expression of signal transducer and activator of transcription 3 (STAT3), a central node of several oncogenic signaling cascades. Suppression of this important transcription factor led to tumor regression via engaging multiple mechanisms, such as antiangiogenic (decrease in VEGF-C expression), antiinflammatory (reduction of TNF-α expression), antiinvasive (decrease in serum MMP-2 and MMP-9 activities) and proapoptotic pathways (increase in caspase-3 levels) [12] (Table 5). Therefore, apigenin can represent a potential radiosensitizer for enhancing the radiation response of solid tumors by triggering multiple cellular pathways for combating radioresistance.

4.4.1.4. Hepatocellular Carcinoma

Apigenin in conjunction with radiation caused an increase in radiation-induced cell killing in Reuber H35 rat hepatoma cells, by suppressing repair of radiation-induced DNA damage and reducing the rate of cell repopulation. This radioenhancing action of apigenin revealed only when apigenin was applied after irradiation for until 24 h [84] (Table 5). Further studies are needed to ascertain whether this radiosensitizing effect of apigenin observed in rat liver tumor cells will be reproducible also in human hepatocellular carcinomas.

4.4.2. Luteolin

Luteolin is a flavonoid isolated from numerous different plants, including edible plants and medicinal herbs. This flavone can be found in a wide range of fruits and vegetables, such as celery, perilla leaf and green pepper, but also in chamomile tea [4, 13, 34] (Table 1).

4.4.2.1. Non-Small Cell Lung Cancer

Pretreatment with luteolin (20 μM, 30 μM) for 6 h was able to potentiate radiation-induced cell killing in two human non-small cell lung cancer cell lines, NCI-H460 and NCI-H1299. Luteolin in combination with ionizing radiation triggered activation of p38 MAPK, promoted generation of ROS, and enhanced apoptotic cell death accompanied by downregulation of Bcl-2 and activation of caspases-3, -8 and -9. As NCI-H460 cells express wild-type p53 and PTEN and NCI-H1299 cells are p53- and PTEN-null, radioenhancing action of luteolin was independent on p53 and PTEN status in malignant lung cells. In addition, luteolin could behave as a potent radiosensitizer also in NCI-H460 xenograft tumor bearing mice, leading to a significant delay of tumor growth and increase in the proportion of apoptotic cells [4] (Table 5). Thus, luteolin could potentially sensitize human non-small cell lung tumors to radiotherapy; the design of clinical trials is highly warranted.

4.4.2.2. Oral Cancer

Luteolin restored sensitivity to ionizing radiation in cancer stem cells (CSCs) derived from two human oral squamous cell carcinoma lines, GNM and SAS. Combined treatment with luteolin and radiation revealed synergistic inhibitory activity on clonogenicity and invasiveness of oral CSCs, probably through inactivation of interleukin-6 (IL-6)/STAT3 signaling by luteolin [34] (Table 5). As CSCs or tumor-initiating cells could drive tumor radioresistance, development of novel strategies which target this subpopulation of malignant cells might be useful for radiosensitization of human tumors.

4.4.2.3. Gastric Cancer

Gastric cancer is the fifth most common cancer type of men and women, with an estimated 1 033 701 new cases in 2018 worldwide [1]. Its incidence is especially high in South Korea, Asia, South America and Eastern Europe [13].

Pretreatment with luteolin (20 μM) for 24 h enhanced radiation-induced inhibition of clonogenic survival of SGC-7901 human gastric cancer cells. This radiosensitizing effect of luteolin was achieved through inhibition of Akt activity, leading to an increase in radiation-induced apoptotic death associated with downregulation of Bcl-2, activation of caspases-3 and -9, and release of cytochrome c from mitochondria into the cytosol. In addition, luteolin in conjunction with radiation caused a significant suppression of prostaglandin E2 production, as well as a reduced expression of VEGF and HIF-1α levels. Moreover, luteolin potentiated the response of SGC-7901 tumor bearing mice to ionizing radiation, resulting in significantly smaller tumors with extended growth delay time [13] (Table 5). These *in vitro* and *in vivo* findings show that luteolin might be a promising candidate of radiosensitizer for treatment of human gastric cancers.

Therefore, luteolin can target different intracellular signaling cascades implicated in resistance to radiation and enhance radiotherapeutic efficacy for several human solid tumors, including non-small cell lung cancer, oral squamous cell carcinoma and gastric tumor.

4.4.3. Baicalein

Baicalein is a widely used compound in Chinese medicine, isolated from the root of *Scutellaria baicalensis* Georgi that contains about 5.41% of this flavone. Baicalein is proven to be non-toxic at its pharmacological doses, as 3-9 g root powder of *Scutellaria* was reported to be safe for adults [43] (Table 1). The maximum plasma doses around 110 ng/ml (0.4 μM) have been measured in human subjects after administration of a single dose of 2800 mg baicalein as a chewable tablet [43].

Table 5. Effects of flavones on cancer radiotherapeutic efficacy

Agent	Cancer site	Biological system	Method	Assay conditions		Effect	Ref.
Apigenin, API	Breast	i.m. inoculation of Ehrlich carcinoma cells into the right thigh muscle of the lower limb of female Swiss albino mouse	Tumor growth analysis	i.p. injection of API (50 mg/kg bw), followed by single whole-body irradiation (6.5 Gy) 30 min later; continuing API treatment for 30 consecutive days	↑	Regression of tumor, reduction of tumor volume. Suppression of NO, increase in caspase-3 and granzyme B; downregulation of STAT3, VEGF-C and TNF-α; decrease in MMPs-2/-9 activity	[12]
	Larynx	s.c. injection of Hep-2 cells into the right forelimb of male athymic nude mouse with a BALB/c background	Tumor growth analysis	i.p. injection of API (100 μg/day for 10 days), irradiation (10 Gy) of the local tumor on day 20	↑	Decrease in tumor size. Reduction of GLUT-1 expression	[54]
	Liver	Reuber H35 rat hepatoma cells	Colony formation	Addition of API for 0.5h before X-ray irradiation (2-8 Gy); continuing incubation for 23.5h	↑	Reduction of cell survival	[84]
	Lung	SQ-5 human lung squamous carcinoma cells	Colony formation	Pretreatment with API (40 μM) for 16h before X-ray irradiation (6 Gy); incubation with API for further 8h	↑	Reduction of survival. Increase in apoptosis (decrease in Bcl-2, PARP cleavage). Increase in WAF1/p21. Radiosensitization in monolayer cultures and spheroids	[65]
Baicalein, BAI	Breast	MCF-7 human breast cancer cells		Treatment with BAI (50 μM) and γ-irradiation (2 Gy)	↑	Synergistic DNA damage. 2.36-fold increase in radiation-induced apoptosis	[43]
Cirsiliol, CIR	Lung	NCI-H460 human non-small cell lung cancer cells	Colony formation	Treatment with CIR (10 μM), exposure to γ-irradiation (2 Gy)	↑	Suppression of proliferation. p53-dependent increase in miR-34a expression leading to downregulation of Notch-1, NF-κB and prosurvival proteins (cIAP1, cIAP2, survivin). Increase in apoptosis, reversal of radiation-induced EMT (increase in E-cadherin; decrease in vimentin, fibronectin)	[28]

Agent	Cancer site	Biological system	Method	Assay conditions	Effect		Ref.
		NCI-H1299 human non-small cell lung cancer cells	Colony formation	Treatment with CIR (10 µM), exposure to γ-irradiation (2 Gy)	↑	Suppression of proliferation. p53-dependent increase in miR-34a expression leading to downregulation of Notch-1, NF-κB and prosurvival proteins (cIAP1, cIAP2, survivin). Increase in apoptosis, reversal of radiation-induced EMT (increase in E-cadherin; decrease in vimentin, fibronectin)	[28]
		Injection of NCI-H1299 cells in the flank of BALB/c athymic nude mice	Tumor growth analysis	i.p. treatment with CIR (200 µg/kg bw) daily for 25 days; irradiation (10 Gy/week) for 3 weeks	↑	Reduction of tumor volume. Increase in miR-34a, decrease in radiation-induced expression of Notch-1, prosurvival proteins (cIAP1, cIAP2, survivin) and EMT-related proteins (vimentin, fibronectin)	[28]
Diosmetin, DIO	Lung	A549/IR human lung cancer cells (radioresistant)	MTS, colony formation	Pretreatment with DIO (10 µM) for 24h before X-ray irradiation (6 Gy)	↑	Inhibition of growth, increase in G1 phase arrest. Restraint of radiation-induced DNA damage repair by inhibiting activated Akt signaling (decrease in phosphorylation of ATM and p53)	[19]
Luteolin, LUT	Lung	NCI-H1299 human non-small cell lung cancer cells	Counting, colony formation	Pretreatment with LUT (20, 30 µM) for 6h before γ-irradiation (2, 3 Gy)	↑	Reduction of survival fraction. Increase in apoptosis (activation of caspases-3/-8/-9, decrease in Bcl-2)	[4]
		NCI-H460 human non-small cell lung cancer cells		Pretreatment with LUT (20, 30 µM) for 6h before γ-irradiation (2, 3 Gy)	↑	Reduction of survival fraction. Increase in apoptosis (activation of caspases-3/-8/-9, decrease in Bcl-2). Increase in p38 phosphorylation and ROS production	[4]
		Injection of NCI-H460 cells to BALB/cAnNCrj-nu/nu mice	Tumor growth analysis	s.c. injection of LUT (10 mg/kg) for 6h before irradiation (5 Gy); repeating this scheme for 3 times at 5-day intervals	↑	Delay in tumor growth. Increase in the number of apoptotic cells	[4]

Table 5. (Continued)

Agent	Cancer site	Biological system	Method	Assay conditions	Effect		Ref.
	Mouth	GNM-CSC cancer stem cells from oral squamous cell carcinoma cells	MTT, colony formation	Treatment with LUT, irradiation with 2-32 Gy	↑	Reduction of survival. Promotion of elimination of colony forming and invasion abilities	[34]
		SAS-CSC cancer stem cells from oral squamous cell carcinoma cells	MTT	Treatment with LUT, irradiation with 2-32 Gy	↑	Reduction of survival. Promotion of elimination of colony forming and invasion abilities	[34]
	Stomach	SGC-7901 human gastric cancer cells	Colony formation	Pretreatment with LUT (20 μM) for 24h before γ-irradiation (8 Gy)	↑	Inhibition of clonogenicity. Increase in intrinsic apoptosis (activation of caspases-3/-9, decrease in Bcl-2, release of cyt c). Reduction of radiation-induced PGE-2 production, downregulation of VEGF and HIF-1α	[13]
		s.c. injection of SGC-7901 cells into the right thigh of BALB/cAnu/nu mice	Tumor growth analysis	s.c. injection of LUT (20 μM/kg) into tumors, irradiation (8 Gy) after 0.5 h	↑	Reduction of tumor volume. Extension of growth delay	[13]
Oroxylin A, ORO	Esophagus	ECA109 human esophageal squamous cell carcinoma cells	Colony formation	Pretreatment with ORO (10, 50 μM) for 24h before X-ray irradiation (2-8 Gy)	↑	Reduction of survival, increase in G2/M arrest and apoptosis	[32]
		TE13 human esophageal squamous cell carcinoma cells		Pretreatment with ORO (10, 50 μM) for 24h before X-ray irradiation (2-8 Gy)	↑	Reduction of survival, increase in G2/M arrest and apoptosis	[32]
Tangeretin, TAN	Stomach	SGC-7901 human gastric cancer cells	Colony formation	Exposure to irradiation (2-8 Gy) and TAN (30 μM) for 24h	↑	Increase in clonogenic death. Decrease in radiation-induced EMT, invasion and migration (decrease in vimentin, N-cadherin; increase in E-cadherin). Inhibition of Notch-1 signaling, elevation of miR-410	[33]

Agent	Cancer site	Biological system	Method	Assay conditions	Effect		Ref.
		s.c. injection of SGC7901 cells into the athymic nude mice	Tumor growth analysis	i.p. treatment with TAN (30 mg/kg) for 3 weeks; exposure to radiation (2 Gy) 5 times a week for 3 weeks	↑	Decrease in tumor size. Attenuation of radiation-induced pulmonary metastasis	[33]
Vicenin-2, VCN	Lung	NCI-H23 non-small cell lung cancer cells	Counting	Pretreatment with VCN (80 μM) for 24h before X-ray radiation (6 Gy)	↑	Lowering of pAkt level. Promotion of proapoptotic environment (decrease in Bcl-2, increase in Bax and caspase-3)	[71]
		NCI-H23 non-small cell lung cancer cells	MTT	Pretreatment with VCN (80 μM) for 24h before X-ray radiation (2-8 Gy)	↑	Reduction of cell survival. Increase in caspase-3 activity and DNA degradation. Decrease in MMP-2 and p21 levels	[74]

4.4.3.1. Breast Cancer

Baicalein (50 µM) significantly enhanced the effect of radiation in MCF-7 human breast cancer cells. Combined treatment with baicalein and radiation led to an elevated extent of DNA damage and promoted apoptotic death as compared to irradiation-only treated cells [43] (Table 5). Thus, baicalein as a non-toxic natural agent is one of the attractive flavonoids relevant for further evaluation as an adjuvant for breast cancer radiotherapy.

4.4.4. Diosmetin

Diosmetin is a monomethylated derivative of luteolin, occurring naturally in legumes, olive leaves, citrus fruits and some medicinal herbs [19] (Table 1).

4.4.4.1. Non-Small Cell Lung Cancer

Diosmetin (10 µM) was shown to act as a potent radiosensitizer for resistant A549 human non-small cell lung cancer cells, A549/IR, by inducing G1 phase cell cycle arrest and strongly inhibiting cell growth. Diosmetin restrained the repair of radiation-induced DNA damage, reducing activation of DNA-PK and ATM and enhancing γ-H2AX foci reflecting accumulation of DNA double-strand breaks. This radioenhancing effect of diosmetin was achieved through suppression of Akt signaling pathway, suggesting that diosmetin could substantially enhance the antitumor action of ionizing radiation [19] (Table 5). Therefore, diosmetin has a promising role in sensitization of lung cancer cells to radiotherapy, especially the radioresistant clones.

4.4.5. Oroxylin A

Oroxylin A is a monomethylated derivative of baicalein (Table 1). Oroxylin A is an important bioactive component of Chinese traditional medicine, extracted from the root of *Scutellaria baicalensis* Georgi [32].

4.4.5.1. Esophageal Cancer
Pretreatment with oroxylin A (10 µM, 50 µM) for 24 h augmented radiation-induced reduction of cell survival fraction in two human esophageal squamous cell carcinoma cell lines, ECA109 and TE13. Oroxylin A in conjunction with radiation led to a significantly greater proportion of cells in G2/M phase with respective decrease in the expression of cyclin B1 and Cdc2, and resulted in a higher apoptosis rate as compared to the treatment with either modality alone [32] (Table 5). These data show that oroxylin A could be a promising radiosensitizer for treatment of esophageal squamous cell carcinoma.

4.4.6. Cirsiliol

Cirsiliol is a dimethylated derivative of luteolin (Table 1).

4.4.6.1. Non-Small Cell Lung Cancer
Exposure to cirsiliol (10 µM) potentiated radiation-induced inhibition of cell proliferation in two human non-small cell lung cancer cell lines, NCI-H1299 and NCI-H460. Cirsiliol upregulated the expression of tumor-suppressive miR-34a levels, in a p53-dependent manner, directly leading to inhibition of radiation-induced Notch-1 overexpression and thereby suppressing the radioresistance and EMT phenotypes. Thus, Notch-1 as a critical oncogenic node could be involved in the survival of lung tumor cells under irradiation. In detail, reduced expression of Notch-1 by cirsiliol resulted in a downregulation

of NF-κB prosurvival signaling, further promoting apoptotic death by suppressing the levels of antiapoptotic proteins, such as cIAP1, cIAP2 and survivin. In addition, inhibition of Notch-1 expression by cirsiliol attenuated also irradiation-induced EMT, reducing cellular motility and invasiveness through increasing E-cadherin and decreasing vimentin and fibronectin levels. As a result, cirsiliol effectively promoted radiosensitivity in lung cancer cells *in vitro*. Furthermore, cirsiliol in conjunction with radiation caused a significant reduction of tumor volume in NCI-H1299 xenograft bearing nude mice as compared with mice receiving radiation alone, thus confirming the *in vitro* results on radiosensitizing properties of cirsiliol. Radiation-elevated expressions of Notch-1, antiapoptotic and EMT-related proteins were suppressed by cirsiliol in extracted tumor tissue lysates, showing that radioenhancing effects of cirsiliol were revealed both *in vitro* as well as *in vivo* models [28] (Table 5). Therefore, cirsiliol can act as a novel potent radiosensitizer for treatment of human lung tumors and the design of clinical trials is highly necessitated.

4.4.7. Tangeretin

Tangeretin is a polymethylated flavonoid (pentamethoxyflavone), occurring in the peel of various citrus fruits, such as tangerines (Table 1).

4.4.7.1. Gastric Cancer

Tangeretin (30 μM) promoted the sensitivity of SGC7901 human gastric cancer cells to ionizing radiation, potentiating the radiation-induced decrease in cell viability. Tangeretin in conjunction with radiation caused an upregulation of tumor-suppressive miR-410 levels, further leading to suppression of Notch-1 expression (but not activation) and reversal of EMT. In fact, combined treatment with tangeretin and radiation prevented radiation-induced EMT and restrained invasive and migratory abilities of gastric cancer cells, by reducing the expression of N-cadherin and vimentin and increasing E-cadherin levels. Further *in vivo* studies showed that tangeretin in conjunction with radiation led to a greater decrease in tumor size in SGC7901 xenograft bearing nude mice as compared to the mice treated with radiation alone. Thereat, mice treated with tangeretin and radiation were in considerably better physical condition than their radiation-only treated counterparts. Moreover, tangeretin almost completely suppressed the incidence of radiation-induced pulmonary metastasis [33] (Table 5). These findings reveal that tangeretin might be an important adjuvant agent to attenuate metastatic spread of primary gastric tumors under radiotherapeutic treatment, with Notch-1 as an important pharmacological target. As overexpression of Notch-1 oncogene is commonly induced by irradiation, inhibitors of Notch-1 might be promising adjuvant agents to enhance the radiotherapeutic efficacy in treatment of human cancers.

4.4.8. Vicenin-2

Vicenin-2 is a diglycosylated derivative of apigenin, obtained from *Ocimum sanctum* L. [71, 74] (Table 1).

4.4.8.1. Non-Small Cell Lung Cancer

Pretreatment with vicenin-2 (80 µM) for 24 h augmented radiation-induced cell killing in NCI-H23 human non-small cell lung cancer cells [71, 74]. Vicenin-2 in conjunction with radiation led to a significant decrease in the level of activated Akt (pAkt). Combined treatment with vicenin-2 and radiation further promoted apoptotic death, by downregulating Bcl-2 and Bcl-xL, and upregulating Bax and caspase-3 levels to a greater extent than the treatment with radiation alone [71]. Pre-exposure to vicenin-2 lowered also the expression of MMP-2 in irradiated cells. This radioenhancing effect of vicenin-2 was specific for tumoral cells, being non-toxic and radioprotective to the normal human fibroblasts [74] (Table 5). Therefore, the radiosensitizing potential of vicenin-2 as a natural safe compound deserves further investigations.

4.5. FLAVONOLIGNANS

4.5.1. Silibinin

Flavonolignan silibinin is the main bioactive component of silymarin, an extract that is obtained from the milk thistle [39] (Table 1). It has been stated that blood plasma concentrations up to 100 μM silibinin could be achieved in humans [48].

4.5.1.1. Prostate Cancer

Silibinin (25 μM) enhanced radiation-induced inhibition of colony formation in two human prostate cancer cell lines, DU145 and PC-3, by potentiating and prolonging radiation-induced G2/M phase cell cycle arrest and promoting apoptotic cell death. Concurrently with blocking the cell cycle progression, the expression levels of cyclin B1 and Cdc2 were reduced. In addition, exposure to silibinin in conjunction with radiation induced downregulation of prosurvival factors survivin and proliferating cell nuclear antigen (PCNA). Specifically, in DU145 cells, mechanisms behind this radiosensitizing effect of silibinin involved augmentation of radiation-induced ROS generation and extension of oxidative stress, with a remarkable reduction of the levels of antioxidant enzymes, including SOD, CAT and GST. Addition of silibinin along with radiation further inhibited repair of radiation-induced DNA damage and EGFR signaling, by downregulating ATM and suppressing nuclear translocation of EGFR and DNA-PK, resulting in prolonged presence of γ-H2AX foci. Eventually, silibinin potentiated radiation-induced apoptotic death by attenuating the levels of Bcl-2 antiapoptotic protein [48]. Moreover, combination of silibinin with ionizing radiation led to a marked suppression of radiation-induced invasion and migration in both DU145 and PC-3 cells, with a decrease in MMP-2 activity. In DU145 cells, silibinin strongly inhibited radiation-induced proangiogenic (VEGF, iNOS), migratory (MMP-2) and EMT-related proteins (N-cadherin, vimentin, uPA). This radiosensitizing effect was driven by attenuating radiation-activated prosurvival signaling, including Akt, ERK1/2 and STAT3, by silibinin [45]. However, in radioresponsive 22Rv1 human prostate cancer cells, no ability of silibinin to further enhance radiotherapeutic response was noticed [48].

In vivo conditions, combined treatment with oral silibinin and radiation led to a strong decrease in tumor burden and inhibition of tumor growth in DU145 xenograft bearing nude mice, with a higher proportion of apoptotic cells and reduced repair of DNA damage as compared to the mice treated with irradiation alone. Moreover, addition of silibinin in conjunction with ionizing radiation rescued the mice from radiation-induced systemic toxicity and hematopoietic injury [48] (Table 6). Thus, silibinin functions as a potent radiosensitizer for human prostate tumors by targeting multiple signaling pathways implicated in development of radioresistance. Further clinical trials using this non-toxic natural flavonolignan are highly justified to translate these promising preclinical findings to actual clinical benefits for prostate cancer patients.

4.5.1.2. Bladder Cancer

Bladder cancer is the second leading cause of mortality from genitourinary malignancy in men [39]. In 2018, 549 393 new bladder cancer cases were estimated to occur worldwide [1].

Silibinin (40 μM, 60 μM) augmented radiation-induced growth inhibition in invasive MB49-I murine bladder cancer cells, but not in non-invasive MB49 murine bladder cancer cells. This radioenhancing effect of silibinin was achieved through enhancement of oxidative stress, and inhibition of radiation-induced survival pathways, NF-κB and PI3K/Akt. Also, addition of silibinin along with ionizing radiation led to a decrease in survivin expression. These *in vitro* findings were further confirmed in *in vivo* conditions, showing that silibinin potentiated radiotherapeutic response and improved overall survival of mice harboring invasive MB49-I murine tumors, but not non-invasive MB49 xenografts [39] (Table 6). Thus, silibinin can inhibit radiation-activated prosurvival pathways in invasive bladder tumors, thereby overcoming radioresistance phenomenon. Further studies with human bladder cancer cells, both invasive and non-invasive, are required to evaluate the chances for development of silibinin as a radiosensitizing agent for human bladder tumors.

4.5.1.3. Non-Small Cell Lung Cancer

Silibinin was shown to potentiate radiation-induced suppression of clonogenic survival in A549 human non-small cell lung cancer cells [48] (Table 6). Further preclinical studies are needed to unravel mechanistic details behind this radiosensitizing effect of silibinin.

Altogether, silibinin could target radiation-induced prosurvival pathways and improve radiotherapeutic response in several human tumors, including prostate, bladder and lung cancers.

4.6. CHALCONES

4.6.1. Isoliquiritigenin

Isoliquiritigenin is a natural chalcone-type flavonoid, occurring in licorice, shallots and bean sprouts [8, 59] (Table 1).

Table 6. Effects of flavonolignans (silibinin) on cancer radiotherapeutic efficacy

Agent	Cancer site	Biological system	Method	Assay conditions	Effect		Ref.
Silibinin, SIL	Bladder	MB49 murine bladder cancer cells (non-invasive)	MTS, colony formation	Pretreatment with SIL (40, 60 μM) for 24h before γ-irradiation (2, 4, 6 Gy)	~	No effect on radiation-induced growth inhibition	[39]
		s.c. injection of MB49 cells into the left flank of C57BL/6J mice	Tumor growth analysis	Treatment with SIL (400 mg/kg) via gavage for 5 days/week; irradiation (3 Gy) as 6 factions (3 fractions/week)	~	No effect on radiation-induced tumor growth inhibition and survival improvement of mice	[39]
		MB49-I murine bladder cancer cells (invasive)	MTS, colony formation	Pretreatment with SIL (40, 60 μM) for 24h before γ-irradiation (2, 4, 6 Gy)	↑	Improvement of growth inhibition. Decrease in radiation-induced NF-κB activation, survivin and pAkt levels. Increase in oxidative stress	[39]
		s.c. injection of MB49-I cells into the left flank of C57BL/6J mice	Tumor growth analysis	Treatment with SIL (400 mg/kg) via gavage for 5 days/week; irradiation (3 Gy) as 6 factions (3 fractions/week)	↑	Increase in radiation-induced tumor growth inhibition. Improvement of mice survival	[39]
	Lung	A549 human lung cancer cells	Colony formation	Treatment with γ-irradiation (2.5-10 Gy) and SIL (25 μM)	↑	Inhibition of colony formation	[48]
	Prostate	22Rv1 human prostate cancer cells (radio-responsive)	Colony formation	Treatment with γ-irradiation (2.5-10 Gy) and SIL (25 μM)	~	No effect on radiosensitivity	[48]
		DU145 human prostate cancer cells		Treatment with γ-irradiation (5 Gy) and SIL (25 μM)	↑	Inhibition of radiation-induced migration and invasion. Decrease in MMP-2 activity; downregulation of radiation-induced Akt, Erk1/2 and Stat-3 pathways. Reversal of radiation-induced E-cadherin decrease; vimentin, N-cadherin, iNOS, uPA, VEGF, eNOS, MMP-2 increase	[45]

Table 6. (Continued)

Agent	Cancer site	Biological system	Method	Assay conditions	Effect		Ref.
		DU145 human prostate cancer cells	Colony formation	Treatment with γ-irradiation (2.5-10 Gy) and SIL (25 µM)	↑	Inhibition of colony formation. Increase in G2/M arrest and apoptosis (decrease in Bcl-2). Downregulation of survival factors (PCNA, survivin). Increase in ROS. Inhibition of DNA repair, suppression of radiation-induced nuclear translocation of DNA-PK leading to increased number of γ-H2AX foci	[48]
		Injection of DU145 cells into the right flank of athymic nu/nu male nude mice	Tumor growth analysis	Oral treatment with SIL (200 mg/kg bw/day), immediately followed by the first dose of radiation (2.5 Gy); continuation of SIL for 5 days/week. Each irradiation fraction (6 times) separated by 2 days	↑	Suppression of tumor growth, decrease in tumor volume and weight. Inhibition of DNA repair, increase in apoptosis	[48]
		PC-3 human prostate cancer cells	Colony formation	Treatment with γ-irradiation (2.5-10 Gy) and SIL (25 µM)	↑	Inhibition of colony formation. Increase in G2/M arrest (decrease in Cyclin B1 and Cdc2) and apoptosis (decrease in Bcl-2). Downregulation of survival factors (PCNA, survivin)	[48]
		PC-3 human prostate cancer cells		Treatment with γ-irradiation (5 Gy) and SIL (25 µM)	↑	Inhibition of radiation-induced migration and invasion. Decrease in MMP-2 activity	[45]

4.6.1.1. Hepatocellular Carcinoma

Pre-exposure to isoliquiritigenin (39 μM) augmented radiation-induced inhibition of cell growth and survival in HepG2 human liver cancer cells, by causing redox imbalance. Isoliquiritigenin exerted dual action on cellular redox status, behaving as a natural antioxidant and leading to reductive stress within the first few hours following its administration. To adapt to this state and maintain redox equilibrium, cells reduced their Nrf2 levels and downregulated Nrf2-dependent antioxidant system. This suppression of antioxidant defense was achieved at 6 h after isoliquiritigenin addition, resulting in production of excessive endogenous ROS and triggering serious oxidative stress. Thus, pretreatment with isoliquiritigenin for 6 h induced cells with attenuated antioxidative capacity, further contributing to exacerbation of radiation-induced oxidative damage to malignant cells and thereby potentiating the radiosensitivity. Combined treatment with isoliquiritigenin and radiation resulted in a significant increase in DNA double-strand breaks and enhanced apoptosis with downregulation of Bcl-2 and upregulation of Bax levels as compared to the cells exposed to ionizing radiation alone [8, 59]. In addition, intraperitoneal administration of isoliquiritigenin for 6 h before irradiation led to a significantly inhibited tumor growth in HepG2 xenografts bearing nude mice as compared to the radiation-only treated counterparts, suggesting that isoliquiritigenin can augment the radiotherapeutic efficacy both *in vitro* as well as *in vivo* hepatoma models [8] (Table 7). Thus, antioxidant isoliquiritigenin could act as a potent radiosensitizer for human liver tumors through behaving as a strong prooxidant. Thereat, exposure duration to natural radiosensitizers might be a critical factor to disturbing the redox status and augmenting radiosensitivity. For isoliquiritigenin, pretreatment for 6 h seemed to be reasonable for switching from antioxidant to prooxidant properties in human liver tumor cells.

4.6.2. Xanthohumol

Xanthohumol as a prenylated chalcone is the principal flavonoid in hops [57] (Table 1).

4.6.2.1. Breast Cancer
Pretreatment with xanthohumol (10 μM) for 24 h enhanced the radiation-induced cell death in MCF-7 human breast cancer cells, but restored the susceptibility to radiotherapy also in doxorubicin-resistant subline, MCF-7/ADR, a p53 mutant line. Thereat, the radiosensitizing ability of xanthohumol was much more prominent in drug-resistant MCF-7/ADR cells than in the parent breast cancer cells. In MCF-7/ADR cells, xanthohumol in combination with radiation resulted in a complete suppression of activated STAT3 levels, and significantly reduced also EGFR levels. Suppression of STAT3 activity by xanthohumol further led to a synergistic increase in death receptors (DRs)-4 and -5 expression, and reduced the levels of antiapoptotic proteins, such as Bcl-xL, survivin and XIAP. As a result, combined treatment with xanthohumol and radiation potentiated radiation-induced apoptotic death in cross-resistant breast cancer cells [57] (Table 7). Therefore, xanthohumol plus radiation holds a noteworthy potential as an effective anti-breast cancer strategy, especially for treatment of drug-resistant clones.

4.6.2.2. Colon Cancer
Pre-exposure to xanthohumol (10 μM) for 24 h was shown to augment the radiosensitivity of HT-29 human colon cancer cells [57] (Table 7). Molecular mechanisms behind this radiosensitization need further preclinical studies.

4.7. ROTENOIDS

4.7.1. Deguelin

Deguelin is a natural flavonoid compound, present in plants of the *Mundulea sericea* (Willd.) A. Chev. family. Deguelin has been proven to be safe for humans [55] (Table 1).

4.7.1.1. Breast Cancer

Pretreatment with very low doses of deguelin (10 nM) for 48 h augmented radiation-induced decrease in clonogenic survival of MDA-MB-231 human breast cancer cells. Combined treatment with deguelin and ionizing radiation caused a significant decrease in expression of radiation-induced activated Akt level (pAkt) and downregulated survivin, thereby leading to potentiation of apoptotic death, associated with markedly increased caspase-3 cleavage. Additionally, deguelin along with irradiation resulted in an enhanced number of cells blocked in the G2/M phase of cell cycle as compared to the treatment with either single modality, altogether resulting in an enhanced sensitivity of cells to ionizing radiation [55] (Table 8). Thus, deguelin could be a potent radiosensitizer for more efficient treatment of human breast tumors. Further studies with molecularly different human breast cancer cells and *in vivo* animal assays are needed to put these preclinical findings into real clinical practice.

4.7.2. Rotenone

Rotenone, the first described natural rotenoid, can be found in several tropical and subtropical plant species (Table 1).

Table 7. Effects of chalcones on cancer radiotherapeutic efficacy

Agent	Cancer site	Biological system	Method	Assay conditions	Effect		Ref.
Isoliquiritigenin, ISO	Liver	HepG2 human liver cancer cells	Counting, colony formation	Pretreatment with ISO (10 μg/ml) for 6h before X-ray irradiation (4 Gy)	↑	Inhibition of proliferation and clonogenic potential. Increase in apoptosis (decrease in Bcl-2/Bax ratio). Decrease in radiation-induced Nrf2 activation, increase in Nox2 expression and ROS; exacerbation of oxidative damage	[59]
		HepG2 human liver cancer cells	Colony formation	Pretreatment with ISO (10 μg/ml) for 6h before X-ray irradiation (4 Gy)	↑	Reduction of clonogenic potential. Increase in DNA damage and apoptosis. Induction of oxidative stress through inhibition of Nrf2-antioxidant pathway	[8]
		s.c. injection of HepG2 cells at the back space of male athymic BALB/c nude mice	Tumor growth analysis	i.p. treatment with ISO (10 mg/kg) for 6h before X-ray irradiation (4 Gy)	↑	Inhibition of tumor growth, decrease in tumor weight	[8]
Xanthohumol, XAN	Breast	MCF-7 human breast cancer cells	MTT	Pretreatment with XAN (10 μM) for 24h before γ-irradiation (10 Gy)	↑	Increase in radiation-induced cell death; decrease in Bcl-xL, increase in DR4 and DR5 levels	[57]
		MCF-7/ADR human breast cancer cells (doxorubicin-resistant)		Pretreatment with XAN (10 μM) for 24h before γ-irradiation (10 Gy)	↑	Increase in radiation-induced cell death. Suppression of STAT3 activity; decrease in Bcl-xL, XIAP, survivin, EGFR levels; increase in DR4 and DR5	[57]
	Colon	HT-29 human colon cancer cells	MTT	Pretreatment with XAN (10 μM) for 24h before γ-irradiation (10 Gy)	↑	Increase in radiation-induced cell death	[57]

Table 8. Effects of rotenoids on cancer radiotherapeutic efficacy

Agent	Cancer site	Biological system	Method	Assay conditions	Effect		Ref.
Deguelin, DEG	Breast	MDA-MB-231 human breast cancer cells	Colony formation	Pretreatment with DEG (10 nM) for 48h before irradiation (3 Gy)	↑	Decrease in clonogenic survival. Increase in G2/M arrest and apoptosis (cleavage of caspase-3). Suppression of pAkt and survivin levels	[55]
Rotenone, ROT	Liver	HepG2 human hepatoma cells	SRB	Pretreatment with ROT (0.5 µM) before X-ray irradiation (2, 4, 8 Gy)	↑	Reduction of cell population. Increase in apoptosis	[51]

4.7.2.1. Hepatocellular Carcinoma

Pretreatment with rotenone (0.5 µM) augmented the response of HepG2 human liver cancer cells to ionizing radiation, by enhancing radiation-induced inhibition of cell proliferation and strengthening the extent of apoptotic death [51] (Table 8). The exact cellular mechanisms behind this radiosensitizing effect of rotenone are still waiting to be unraveled.

Chapter 5

CONCLUSION AND FURTHER CHALLENGES

Emerging evidence suggests that structurally different flavonoids, which are safe dietary components, might serve as potent agents for enhancing the radiotherapeutic efficacy in the treatment of several human cancer types, including such common malignancies as prostate, breast, lung and colorectal tumors. The findings compiled in this book convincingly demonstrate the radiosensitizing capability of soy isoflavones, quercetin, apigenin, luteolin, silibinin and several other frequently found natural flavonoids in various preclinical tumor models, both *in vitro* and *in vivo*. These results might be valuable in developing novel more efficient therapeutic regimens for patients undergoing radiotherapy, especially for resistant tumors.

Complementary approach using natural non-toxic dietary flavonoids in combination with radiotherapy could contribute to enhancement of clinical outcomes by potentiating the local control and debulking of tumor sites caused by irradiation. Additionally, such interventions can mitigate also the adverse effects of irradiation on surrounding normal tissues in the field of irradiation, due to making decrease in irradiation doses feasible for achieving desired cancer cell killing. Therefore, the use of flavonoids as adjuvant agents for radiotherapy might confer improvement of survival and quality of life of cancer patients.

The radiosensitizing effects of flavonoids can be achieved through inhibiting multiple cellular prosurvival pathways activated by irradiation. Such central target molecules for flavonoids include APE1/Ref-1, NF-κB, HIF-1α, Nrf2, Akt, Erk1/2, STAT3, Notch-1. Downregulation of these pathways can disrupt DNA repair processes, induce blockade of cell cycle progression and proliferation, drive malignant cells to apoptotic death and control metastatic spread. Thereat, different mixtures of flavonoids, such as soy isoflavones or green tea extracts, can be even more potent in enhancing the response of tumoral cells to ionizing radiation as compared to the pure flavonoids administered alone. The safety profile of these natural agents is not less important in combating radioresistance, with minimal undesired reactions. Nevertheless, the exact action of flavonoids added along with radiation treatment depends on several factors, including tumor types and cellular characteristics, but also concentrations of flavonoids and their exposure durations. Activities through other, currently unreported, mechanisms cannot be excluded.

Although flavonoids are generally known as potent natural antioxidant agents, many of them can behave also as prooxidants under certain conditions and thereby contribute to radiosensitization. Such biased action of flavonoids in modulating the redox status is a valuable asset, enhancing radiotherapeutic efficacy in malignant cells and simultaneously protecting nearby normal tissues from radiation injury by exerting antioxidant and antiinflammatory activities. The radioprotective action of flavonoids on normal healthy cells is not the focus of this book; however, it is a critical issue considering the aim to develop combinatorial strategies for clinical application in the future.

The use of non-toxic dietary flavonoids to augment the efficacy of radiotherapy is promising for the design of novel clinical strategies for the treatment of human cancers. Nevertheless, there are still a number of issues waiting to be addressed first.

- The exact cellular mechanisms and molecular targets involved in radiosensitization effects of flavonoids require detailed unravelling and further in-depth mechanistic studies, both *in vitro* and *in vivo* preclinical models.
- The current research has conducted in a rather restricted choice of model systems. Therefore, additional works in molecularly different cancerous cells are important to elucidate the generality and specificity issues.
- Further preclinical studies should address the questions related to appropriate dosage, timing and exposure duration of flavonoids in conjunction with radiation to find the optimal protocol for designing clinical trials.
- Clinical trials are highly needed to translate the promising preclinical findings into practice and exploit the radioenhancing capability of flavonoids for patients suffering from different cancers, especially radioresistant tumors.
- In parallel to the implementation of clinical trials, safety profile of certain natural flavonoids should be (re-)confirmed.
- Additionally, only a limited selection of flavonoids has been studied to date concerning their potential radiomodulatory properties and thus, more investigations with structurally different flavonoids are encouraged. In fact, no studies are presently available in combining radiation treatment with flavanones present in citrus fruits or anthocyanidins occurring in various berries.
- Last but not least, as it is well known that dietary flavonoids undergo excessive metabolic conversion following their oral ingestion, potential radiomodulating action and relative contribution of metabolic derivatives to the radioenhancing effects observed with parent flavonoids should also be elucidated in the future.

However, despite the numerous compelling radiosensitizing effects described in literature and compiled in this book, there are some reports available also about the undesired antagonistic action of flavonoids in human malignant cells when applied in combination with ionizing radiation. Pure genistein could upregulate radiation-induced activation of prosurvival molecules Akt and ERK1/2 in human colorectal cancer cells [68], and enhance survival fraction of irradiated glioblastoma cells [77] and myeloid leukemia cells [52, 87] at lower micromolar doses achievable through oral intake. Also, EGCG behaved as a free radical scavenger and suppressed radiation-induced cell killing in human prostate cancer cells [76], and attenuated radiotoxicity in human oral cancer cells [89]. These findings point to some contradictions in the use of antioxidants along with radiotherapy, highlighting the necessity for further research. Moreover, although being reported in *in vitro* assays, these data still warn patients undergoing radiotherapy against the use of flavonoid-rich dietary supplements on their own initiative.

In summary, the ultimate goal of *in vitro* and *in vivo* studies combining flavonoids and ionizing radiation is to identify specific radioenhancing agent(s) for malignant tissues with no damaging (and preferably protecting) action on surrounding normal cells for successful application in the clinical settings in the future. For this purpose, fine tuning of all aspects, in particular the appropriate dosage schedules, is crucial. With no doubt, flavonoids represent potent radiosensitizers to augment radiation-induced cancer cell killing and probably it is only a matter of time, when these natural non-toxic agents will be routinely used as adjuvant agents for radiotherapeutic treatment of human tumors, to enhance the clinical outcome, prolong survival time and improve quality of life of patients. Therefore, it is possible that the actual therapeutic capacity of natural flavonoids manifests in complementary strategies together with conventional anticancer treatment modalities, such as radiotherapy, rather than their own cytotoxic activities.

REFERENCES

[1] Bray F, Ferlay J, Soerjomataram I, Siegel RL, Torre LA, Jemal A. Global cancer statistics 2018: GLOBOCAN estimates of incidence of mortality worldwide for 36 cancers in 185 countries. *CA Cancer J Clin* 2018; 68: 394-424.

[2] Madia F, Worth A, Whelan M, Corvi R. Carcinogenicity assessment: Addressing the challenges of cancer and chemicals in the environment. *Environ Int* 2019; 128: 417-29.

[3] Gong C, Yang Z, Zhang L, Wang Y, Gong W, Liu Y. Quercetin suppresses DNA double-strand break repair and enhances the radiosensitivity of human ovarian cancer cells via p53-dependent endoplasmic reticulum stress pathway. *Onco Targets Ther* 2017; 11: 17-27.

[4] Cho HJ, Ahn KC, Choi JY, Hwang SG, Kim WJ, Um HD, Park JK. Luteolin acts as a radiosensitizer in non-small cell lung cancer cells by enhancing apoptotic cell death through activation of a p38/ROS/caspase cascade. *Int J Oncol* 2015; 46: 1149-58.

[5] Kuo WT, Tsai YC, Wu HC, Ho YJ, Chen YS, Yao CH, Yao CH. Radiosensitization of non-small cell lung cancer by kaempferol. *Oncol Rep* 2015; 34: 2351-6.

[6] Nambiar D, Rajamani P, Singh RP. Effects of phytochemicals on ionization radiation-mediated carcinogenesis and cancer therapy. *Mutat Res* 2011; 728: 139-57.

[7] Lawenda BD, Smith DE, Xu L, Niemierko A, Silverstein JR, Boucher Y, Kashiwagi S, Held KD, Jain RK, Loeffler JS, Eisenberg DM, Blumberg JB. Do the dietary supplements epigallocatechin gallate or vitamin e cause a radiomodifying response on tumors in vivo? A pilot study with murine breast carcinoma. *J Soc Integr Oncol* 2007; 5: 11-7.

[8] Sun C, Wang ZH, Liu XX, Yang LN, Wang Y, Liu Y, Mao AH, Liu YY, Zhou X, Di CX, Gan L, Zhang H. Disturbance of redox status enhances radiosensitivity of hepatocellular carcinoma. *Am J Cancer Res* 2015; 5: 1368-81.

[9] Sak K. Cytotoxicity of dietary flavonoids on different human cancer types. *Pharmacogn Rev* 2014; 8: 122-46.

[10] Sak K, Everaus H. Multi-target cytotoxic actions of flavonoids in blood cancer cells. *Asian Pac J Cancer Prev* 2015; 16: 4843-7.

[11] Liu X, Sun C, Jin X, Li P, Ye F, Zhao T, Gong L, Li Q. Genistein enhances the radiosensitivity of breast cancer cells via G2/M cell cycle arrest and apoptosis. *Molecules* 2013; 18: 13200-17.

[12] Medhat AM, Azab KS, Said MM, El Fatih NM, El Bakary NM. Antitumor and radiosensitizing synergistic effects of apigenin and cryptotanshinone against solid Ehrlich carcinoma in female mice. *Tumour Biol* 2017; 39: 1010428317728480.

[13] Zhang Q, Wan L, Guo Y, Cheng N, Cheng W, Sun Q, Zhu J. Radiosensitization effect of luteolin on human gastric cancer SGC-7901 cells. *J Biol Regul Homeost Agents* 2009; 23: 71-8.

[14] Sarkar FH, Li Y. Using chemopreventive agents to enhance the efficacy of cancer therapy. *Cancer Res* 2006; 66: 3347-50.

[15] Lin C, Yu Y, Zhao HG, Yang A, Yan H, Cui Y. Combination of quercetin with radiotherapy enhances tumor radiosensitivity in vitro and in vivo. *Radiother Oncol* 2012; 104: 395-400.

[16] Hillman GG, Singh-Gupta V. Soy isoflavones sensitize cancer cells to radiotherapy. *Free Radic Biol Med* 2011; 51: 289-98.

[17] Hong J, Zhang Z, Lv W, Zhang M, Chen C, Yang S, Li S, Zhang L, Han D, Zhang W. Icaritin synergistically enhances the radiosensitivity of 4T1 breast cancer cells. *PLoS One* 2013; 8: e71347.

[18] Elbaz HA, Lee I, Antwih DA, Liu K, Hüttemann M, Zielske SP. Epicatechin stimulates mitochondrial activity and selectively sensitizes cancer cells to radiation. *PLoS One* 2014; 9: e88322.

[19] Xu Z, Yan Y, Xiao L, Dai S, Zeng S, Qian L, Wang L, Yang X, Xiao Y, Gong Z. Radiosensitizing effect of diosmetin on radioresistant lung cancer cells via Akt signaling pathway. *PLoS One* 2017; 12: e0175977.

[20] Raffoul JJ, Wang Y, Kucuk O, Forman JD, Sarkar FH, Hillman GG. Genistein inhibits radiation-induced activation of NF-kappaB in prostate cancer cells promoting apoptosis and G2/M cell cycle arrest. *BMC Cancer* 2006; 6: 107.

[21] Raffoul JJ, Banerjee S, Singh-Gupta V, Knoll ZE, Fite A, Zhang H, Abrams J, Sarkar FH, Hillman GG. Down-regulation of apurinic/apyrimidinic endonuclease 1/redox factor-1 expression by soy isoflavones enhances prostate cancer radiotherapy in vitro and in vivo. *Cancer Res* 2007; 67: 2141-9.

[22] Hillman GG, Wang Y, Kucuk O, Che M, Doerge DR, Yudelev M, Joiner MC, Marples B, Forman JD, Sarkar FH. Genistein potentiates inhibition of tumor growth by radiation in a prostate cancer orthotopic model. *Mol Cancer Ther* 2004; 3: 1271-9.

[23] Singh-Gupta V, Zhang H, Yunker CK, Ahmad Z, Zwier D, Sarkar FH, Hillman GG. Daidzein effect on hormone refractory prostate cancer in vitro and in vivo compared to genistein and soy extract: potentiation of radiotherapy. *Pharm Res* 2010; 27: 1115-27.

[24] Ahmad IU, Forman JD, Sarkar FH, Hillman GG, Heath E, Vaishampayan U, Cher ML, Andic F, Rossi PJ, Kucuk O. Soy isoflavones in conjunction with radiation therapy in patients with prostate cancer. *Nutr Cancer* 2010; 62: 996-1000.

[25] Singh-Gupta V, Joiner MC, Runyan L, Yunker CK, Sarkar FH, Miller S, Gadgeel SM, Konski AA, Hillman GG. Soy isoflavones augment radiation effect by inhibiting APE1/Ref-1 DNA repair activity in non-small cell lung cancer. *J Thorac Oncol* 2011; 6: 688-98.

[26] Hermann RM, Fest J, Christiansen H, Hille A, Rave-Fränk M, Nitsche M, Gründker C, Viereck V, Jarry H, Schmidberger H. Radiosensitization dependent on p53 function in bronchial carcinoma cells by the isoflavone genistein and estradiol in vitro. *Strahlenther Onkol* 2007; 183: 195-202.

[27] Panat NA, Singh BG, Maurya DK, Sandur SK, Ghaskadbi SS. Troxerutin, a natural flavonoid binds to DNA minor groove and enhances cancer cell killing in response to radiation. *Chem Biol Interact* 2016; 251: 34-44.

[28] Kang J, Kim E, Kim W, Seong KM, Youn H, Kim JW, Kim J, Youn B. Rhamnetin and cirsiliol induce radiosensitization and inhibition of epithelial-mesenchymal transition (EMT) by miR-34a-mediated suppression of Notch-1 expression in non-small cell lung cancer cell lines. *J Biol Chem* 2013; 288: 27343-57.

[29] Hillman GG, Singh-Gupta V, Hoogstra DJ, Abernathy L, Rakowski J, Yunker CK, Rothstein SE, Sarkar FH, Gadgeel S, Konski AA, Lonardo F, Joiner MC. Differential effect of soy isoflavones in enhancing high intensity radiotherapy and protecting lung tissue in a pre-clinical model of lung carcinoma. *Radiother Oncol* 2013; 109: 117-25.

[30] Hillman GG, Singh-Gupta V, Runyan L, Yunker CK, Rakowski JT, Sarkar FH, Miller S, Gadgeel SM, Sethi S, Joiner MC, Konski AA. Soy isoflavones radiosensitize lung cancer while mitigating normal tissue injury. *Radiother Oncol* 2011; 101: 329-36.

[31] Zhang B, Fan X, Wang Z, Zhu W, Li J. Alpinumisoflavone radiosensitizes esophageal squamous cell carcinoma through inducing apoptosis and cell cycle arrest. *Biomed Pharmacother* 2017; 95: 199-206.

[32] Tan C, Qian X, Ge Y, Yang B, Wang F, Guan Z, Cai J. Oroxylin a could be a promising radiosensitizer for esophageal squamous cell carcinoma by inducing G2/M arrest and activating apoptosis. *Pathol Oncol Res* 2017; 23: 323-8.

[33] Zhang X, Zheng L, Sun Y, Wang T, Wang B. Tangeretin enhances radiosensitivity and inhibits the radiation-induced epithelial-

mesenchymal transition of gastric cancer cells. *Oncol Rep* 2015; 34: 302-10.

[34] Tu DG, Lin WT, Yu CC, Lee SS, Peng CY, Lin T, Yu CH. Chemotherapeutic effects of luteolin on radio-sensitivity enhancement and interleukin-6/signal transducer and activator of transcription 3 signaling repression of oral cancer stem cells. *J Formos Med Assoc* 2016; 115: 1032-8.

[35] Yashar CM, Spanos WJ, Taylor DD, Gercel-Taylor C. Potentiation of the radiation effect with genistein in cervical cancer cells. *Gynecol Oncol* 2005; 99: 199-205.

[36] Zhang B, Liu JY, Pan JS, Han SP, Yin XX, Wang B, Hu G. Combined treatment of ionizing radiation with genistein on cervical cancer HeLa cells. *J Pharmacol Sci* 2006; 102: 129-35.

[37] Leu JD, Wang BS, Chiu SJ, Chang CY, Chen CC, Chen FD, Avirmed S, Lee YJ. Combining fisetin and ionizing radiation suppresses the growth of mammalian colorectal cancers in xenograft tumor models. *Oncol Lett* 2016; 12: 4975-82.

[38] Chen WS, Lee YJ, Yu YC, Hsaio CH, Yen JH, Yu SH, Tsai YJ, Chiu SJ. Enhancement of p53-mutant human colorectal cancer cells radiosensitivity by flavonoid fisetin. *Int J Radiat Oncol Biol Phys* 2010; 77: 1527-35.

[39] Prack Mc Cormick B, Langle Y, Belgorosky D, Vanzulli S, Balarino N, Sandes E, Eiján AM. Flavonoid silybin improves the response to radiotherapy in invasive bladder cancer. *J Cell Biochem* 2018; 119: 5402-12.

[40] McLaughlin N, Annabi B, Lachambre MP, Kim KS, Bahary JP, Moumdjian R, Béliveau R. Combined low dose ionizing radiation and green tea-derived epigallocatechin-3-gallate treatment induces human brain endothelial cells death. *J Neurooncol* 2006; 80: 111-21.

[41] Lagerweij T, Hiddingh L, Biesmans D, Crommentuijn MH, Cloos J, Li XN, Kogiso M, Tannous BA, Vandertop WP, Noske DP, Kaspers GJ, Würdinger T, Hulleman E. A chemical screen for medulloblastoma identifies quercetin as a putative radiosensitizer. *Oncotarget* 2016; 7: 35776-88.

[42] McLaughlin N, Annabi B, Bouzeghrane M, Temme A, Bahary JP, Moumdjian R, Béliveau R. The survivin-mediated radioresistant phenotype of glioblastomas is regulated by RhoA and inhibited by the green tea polyphenol (-)-epigallocatechin-3-gallate. *Brain Res* 2006; 1071: 1-9.

[43] Gade S, Gandhi NM. Baicalein inhibits MCF-7 cell proliferation in vitro, induces radiosensitivity, and inhibits hypoxia inducible factor. *J Environ Pathol Toxicol Oncol* 2015; 34: 299-308.

[44] Puthli A, Tiwari R, Mishra KP. Biochanin A enhances the radiotoxicity in colon tumor cells in vitro. *J Environ Pathol Toxicol Oncol* 2013; 32: 189-203.

[45] Nambiar DK, Rajamani P, Singh RP. Silibinin attenuates ionizing radiation-induced pro-angiogenic response and EMT in prostate cancer cells. *Biochem Biophys Res Commun* 2015; 456: 262-8.

[46] Zhang Z, Jin F, Lian X, Li M, Wang G, Lan B, He H, Liu GD, Wu Y, Sun G, Xu CX, Yang ZZ. Genistein promotes ionizing radiation-induced cell death by reducing cytoplasmic Bcl-xL levels in non-small cell lung cancer. *Sci Rep* 2018; 8: 328.

[47] Zhang Y, Wei Y, Zhu Z, Gong W, Liu X, Hou Q, Sun Y, Chai J, Zou L, Zhou T. Icariin enhances radiosensitivity of colorectal cancer cells by suppressing NF-κB activity. *Cell Biochem Biophys* 2014; 69: 303-10.

[48] Nambiar DK, Rajamani P, Deep G, Jain AK, Agarwal R, Singh RP. Silibinin preferentially radiosensitizes prostate cancer by inhibiting DNA repair signaling. *Mol Cancer Ther* 2015; 14: 2722-34.

[49] Vijay M, Sivagami G, Thayalan K, Nalini N. Radiosensitizing potential of rutin against human colon adenocarcinoma HT-29 cells. *Bratisl Lek Listy* 2016; 117: 171-8.

[50] Bando SI, Hatano O, Takemori H, Kubota N, Ohnishi K. Potentiality of syringetin for preferential radiosensitization to cancer cells. *Int J Radiat Biol* 2017; 93: 286-94.

[51] Zhang X, Zhou X, Chen R, Zhang H. Radiosensitization by inhibiting complex I activity in human hepatoma HepG2 cells to X-ray radiation. *J Radiat Res* 2012; 53: 257-63.

[52] Jeong MH, Jin YH, Kang EY, Jo WS, Park HT, Lee JD, Yoo YJ, Jeong SJ. The modulation of radiation-induced cell death by genistein in K562 cells: activation of thymidine kinase 1. *Cell Res* 2004; 14: 295-302.

[53] Tang Q, Ma J, Sun J, Yang L, Yang F, Zhang W, Li R, Wang L, Wang Y, Wang H. Genistein and AG1024 synergistically increase the radiosensitivity of prostate cancer cells. *Oncol Rep* 2018; 40: 579-88.

[54] Bao YY, Zhou SH, Lu ZJ, Fan J, Huang YP. Inhibiting GLUT-1 expression and PI3K/Akt signaling using apigenin improves the radiosensitivity of laryngeal carcinoma in vivo. *Oncol Rep* 2015; 34: 1805-14.

[55] Yi T, Li H, Wang X, Wu Z. Enhancement radiosensitization of breast cancer cells by deguelin. *Cancer Biother Radiopharm* 2008; 23: 355-62.

[56] Enkhbat T, Nishi M, Yoshikawa K, Jun H, Tokunaga T, Takasu C, Kashihara H, Ishikawa D, Tominaga M, Shimada M. Epigallocatechin-3-gallate enhances radiation sensitivity in colorectal cancer cells through Nrf2 activation and autophagy. *Anticancer Res* 2018; 38: 6247-52.

[57] Kang Y, Park MA, Heo SW, Park SY, Kang KW, Park PH, Kim JA. The radio-sensitizing effect of xanthohumol is mediated by STAT3 and EGFR suppression in doxorubicin-resistant MCF-7 human breast cancer cells. *Biochim Biophys Acta* 2013; 1830: 2638-48.

[58] Luttjeboer M, Lafleur MV, Kwidama ZJ, Van Rijn J, Van Den Berg J, Slotman BJ, Kaspers GJ, Cloos J. Strategies for the analysis of in vitro radiation sensitivity and prediction of interaction with potential radiation modifying agents. *Int J Radiat Biol* 2010; 86: 458-66.

[59] Sun C, Zhang H, Ma XF, Zhou X, Gan L, Liu YY, Wang ZH. Isoliquiritigenin enhances radiosensitivity of HepG2 cells via disturbance of redox status. *Cell Biochem Biophys* 2013; 65: 433-44.

[60] Liu X, Sun C, Liu B, Jin X, Li P, Zheng X, Zhao T, Li F, Li Q. Genistein mediates the selective radiosensitizing effect in NSCLC A549 cells via inhibiting methylation of the keap1 gene promoter region. *Oncotarget* 2016; 7: 27267-79.

[61] Liu XX, Sun C, Jin XD, Li P, Zheng XG, Zhao T, Li Q. Genistein sensitizes sarcoma cells in vitro and in vivo by enhancing apoptosis and by inhibiting DSB repair pathways. *J Radiat Res* 2016; 57: 227-37.

[62] Zhang S, Wang L, Liu H, Zhao G, Ming L. Enhancement of recombinant myricetin on the radiosensitivity of lung cancer A549 and H1299 cells. *Diagn Pathol* 2014; 9: 68.

[63] Baatout S, Derradji H, Jacquet P, Mergeay M. Increased radiation sensitivity of an eosinophilic cell line following treatment with epigallocatechin-gallate, resveratrol and curcuma. *Int J Mol Med* 2005; 15: 337-52.

[64] Baatout S, Jacquet P, Derradji H, Ooms D, Michaux A, Mergeay M. Study of the combined effect of X-irradiation and epigallocatechin-gallate (a tea component) on the growth inhibition and induction of apoptosis in human cancer cell lines. *Oncol Rep* 2004; 12: 159-67.

[65] Watanabe N, Hirayama R, Kubota N. The chemopreventive flavonoid apigenin confers radiosensitizing effect in human tumor cells grown as monolayers and spheroids. *J Radiat Res* 2007; 48: 45-50.

[66] Shin JI, Shim JH, Kim KH, Choi HS, Kim JW, Lee HG, Kim BY, Park SN, Park OJ, Yoon DY. Sensitization of the apoptotic effect of gamma-irradiation in genistein-pretreated CaSki cervical cancer cells. *J Microbiol Biotechnol* 2008; 18: 523-31.

[67] Zhang G, Wang Y, Zhang Y, Wan X, Li J, Liu K, Wang F, Liu K, Liu Q, Yang C, Yu P, Huang Y, Wang S, Jiang P, Qu Z, Luan J, Duan H, Zhang L, Hou A, Jin S, Hsieh TC, Wu E. Anti-cancer activities of tea epigallocatechin-3-gallate in breast cancer patients under radiotherapy. *Curr Mol Med* 2012; 12: 163-76.

[68] Gruca A, Krawczyk Z, Szeja W, Grynkiewicz G, Rusin A. Synthetic genistein glycosides inhibiting EGFR phosphorylation enhance the effect of radiation in HCT 116 colon cancer cells. *Molecules* 2014; 19: 18558-73.

[69] Akimoto T, Nonaka T, Ishikawa H, Sakurai H, Saitoh JI, Takahashi T, Mitsuhashi N. Genistein, a tyrosine kinase inhibitor, enhanced radiosensitivity in human esophageal cancer cell lines in vitro:

possible involvement of inhibition of survival signal transduction pathways. *Int J Radiat Oncol Biol Phys* 2001; 50: 195-201.

[70] Garg AK, Buchholz TA, Aggarwal BB. Chemosensitization and radiosensitization of tumors by plant polyphenols. *Antioxid Redox Signal* 2005; 7: 1630-47.

[71] Baruah TJ, Kma L. Vicenin-2 acts as a radiosensitizer of the non-small cell lung cancer by lowering Akt expression. *Biofactors* 2019; 45: 200-10.

[72] Singh-Gupta V, Zhang H, Banerjee S, Kong D, Raffoul JJ, Sarkar FH, Hillman GG. Radiation-induced HIF-1alpha cell survival pathway is inhibited by soy isoflavones in prostate cancer cells. *Int J Cancer* 2009; 124: 1675-84.

[73] Raffoul JJ, Sarkar FH, Hillman GG. Radiosensitization of prostate cancer by soy isoflavones. *Curr Cancer Drug Targets* 2007; 7: 759-65.

[74] Baruah TJ, Sharan RN, Kma L. Vicenin-2: a potential radiosensitizer of non-small cell lung cancer cells. *Mol Biol Rep* 2018; 45: 1219-25.

[75] Taghizadeh B, Ghavami L, Nikoofar A, Goliaei B. Equol as a potent radiosensitizer in estrogen receptor-positive and -negative human breast cancer cell lines. *Breast Cancer* 2015; 22: 382-90.

[76] Thomas F, Holly JM, Persad R, Bahl A, Perks CM. Green tea extract (epigallocatechin-3-gallate) reduces efficacy of radiotherapy on prostate cancer cells. *Urology* 2011; 78: e475.e15-21.

[77] Atefeh Z, Vahid C, Hasan N, Saeed A, Mahnaz H. Combination treatment of glioblastoma by low-dose radiation and genistein. *Curr Radiopharm* 2016; 9: 258-63.

[78] Yan SX, Ejima Y, Sasaki R, Zheng SS, Demizu Y, Soejima T, Sugimura K. Combination of genistein with ionizing radiation on androgen-independent prostate cancer cells. *Asian J Androl* 2004; 6: 285-90.

[79] Wang Y, Raffoul JJ, Che M, Doerge DR, Joiner MC, Kucuk O, Sarkar FH, Hillman GG. Prostate cancer treatment is enhanced by genistein in vitro and in vivo in a syngeneic orthotopic tumor model. *Radiat Res* 2006; 166: 73-80.

[80] Hillman GG, Forman JD, Kucuk O, Yudelev M, Maughan RL, Rubio J, Layer A, Tekyi-Mensah S, Abrams J, Sarkar FH. Genistein potentiates the radiation effect on prostate carcinoma cells. *Clin Cancer Res* 2001; 7: 382-90.

[81] Hillman GG, Wang Y, Che M, Raffoul JJ, Yudelev M, Kucuk O, Sarkar FH. Progression of renal cell carcinoma is inhibited by genistein and radiation in an orthotopic model. *BMC Cancer* 2007; 7: 4.

[82] Raffoul JJ, Banerjee S, Che M, Knoll ZE, Doerge DR, Abrams J, Kucuk O, Sarkar FH, Hillman GG. Soy isoflavones enhance radiotherapy in a metastatic prostate cancer model. *Int J Cancer* 2007; 120: 2491-8.

[83] Hermann RM, Wolff HA, Jarry H, Thelen P, Gruendker C, Rave-Fraenk M, Schmidberger H, Christiansen H. In vitro studies on the modification of low-dose hyper-radiosensitivity in prostate cancer cells by incubation with genistein and estradiol. *Radiat Oncol* 2008; 3: 19.

[84] van Rijn J, van den Berg J. Flavonoids as enhancers of x-ray-induced cell damage in hepatoma cells. *Clin Cancer Res* 1997; 3: 1775-9.

[85] Pozsgai E, Bellyei S, Cseh A, Boronkai A, Racz B, Szabo A, Sumegi B, Hocsak E. Quercetin increases the efficacy of glioblastoma treatment compared to standard chemoradiotherapy by the suppression of PI-3-kinase-Akt pathway. *Nutr Cancer* 2013; 65: 1059-66.

[86] Papazisis KT, Zambouli D, Kimoundri OT, Papadakis ES, Vala V, Geromichalos GD, Voyatzi S, Markala D, Destouni E, Boutis L, Kortsaris AH. Protein tyrosine kinase inhibitor, genistein, enhances apoptosis and cell cycle arrest in K562 cells treated with gamma-irradiation. *Cancer Lett* 2000; 160: 107-13.

[87] Jeong SJ, Jin YH, Moon CW, Bae HR, Yoo YH, Lee HS, Lee SH, Lim YJ, Lee JD, Jeong MH. Protein tyrosine kinase inhibitors modulate radiosensitivity and radiation-induced apoptosis in K562 cells. *Radiat Res* 2001; 156: 751-60.

[88] Lecumberri E, Dupertuis YM, Mirabell R, Pichard C. Green tea polyphenol epigallocatechin-3-gallate (EGCG) as adjuvant in cancer therapy. *Clin Nutr* 2013; 32: 894-903.

[89] Yamamoto T, Staples J, Wataha J, Lewis J, Lockwood P, Schoenlein P, Rao S, Osaki T, Dickinson D, Kamatani T, Schuster G, Hsu S. Protective effects of EGCG on salivary gland cells treated with gamma-radiation or cis-platinum(II)diammine dichloride. *Anticancer Res* 2004; 24: 3065-73.

ABOUT THE AUTHOR

Katrin Sak
Email: katrin.sak.001@mail.ee

The author of this book, Dr. Katrin Sak, was born in Viljandi, Estonia, in 1975. After studies in the University of Tartu, Estonia, she received a Bachelor`s degree (BSc) in Chemistry in 1996 and a Masters degree (MSc) in Bioorganic Chemistry in 1997. In 2001, she was graduated with a Doctorate degree (PhD) in Bioorganic Chemistry. From 2001-2004, Dr. Sak did postdoctoral research at the Free University of Brussels, Belgium and in 2012, she acquired a diploma in cancer nutrition in the Health Schools Australia.

The major research topics of Dr. Sak involve different anticancer actions of plant-derived flavonoids in diverse malignant systems, engaged cellular target molecules and modulated signaling pathways, besides the metabolic bioconversion of these food polyphenols in the human body and bioactivities of various metabolites. In addition, the scientific activity of Dr. Sak is also focused on the interactions between dietary flavonoids and traditional anticancer treatment modalities, including chemotherapy and radiotherapy.

Dr. Sak is the author of two international monographies *Flavonoids in the Fight against Upper Gastrointestinal Tract Cancers* (Nova Science Publishers, Inc., New York, 2018) and *Plant Flavonoids Affect Cancer Chemotherapeutic Efficacy: A Handbook for Doctors and Patients* (Nova Science Publishers, Inc., New York, 2019). She has published more than 80 articles in international peer-reviewed journals and several chapters in handbooks about nutraceuticals, is the author of the book Food and Cancer (in Estonian, 2013) and numerous popular-scientific articles published in the Estonian health journals. Katrin Sak is the head of the NGO Praeventio.

INDEX

#

5-fluorouracil, 3

A

adenocarcinoma, 31, 45, 50, 73, 79, 116
adjuvant, viii, xi, 2, 7, 17, 57, 58, 62, 63, 65, 67, 75, 80, 90, 93, 106, 108, 119
adverse reactions, viii, xi, 2
androgen, xiii, 27, 29, 33, 34, 35, 37, 38, 41, 42, 43, 53, 58, 60, 117
angiogenesis, 14
antioxidant, xiii, 7, 8, 18, 19, 45, 56, 58, 79, 94, 99, 102, 106, 108
apoptosis, xiv, xvi, 6, 8, 9, 10, 11, 13, 15, 27, 28, 29, 30, 31, 33, 34, 35, 37, 45, 46, 52, 53, 56, 58, 59, 60, 62, 64, 68, 69, 70, 72, 73, 74, 82, 86, 87, 88, 91, 98, 99, 102, 103, 110, 111, 112, 116, 118,
apoptotic death, 7, 8, 10, 11, 12, 18, 42, 45, 48, 49, 50, 51, 54, 55, 57, 63, 66, 75, 78, 79, 80, 81, 85, 90, 92, 93, 94, 100, 101, 104, 106
astrocytoma, 59
autophagic death, 45

autophagy, 15, 33, 46, 115

B

berries, 23, 24, 64, 76, 79, 107
bioconversion, 121
bladder cancer, 2, 95, 96, 97, 113
blood brain barrier, 52, 62, 65
blood cancer, 62, 110
brain cancer, 1, 2, 59, 64, 67
breast cancer, 2, 11, 13, 14, 20, 29, 30, 47, 48, 53, 54, 57, 60, 65, 69, 71, 80, 83, 86, 90, 100, 101, 102, 103, 110, 111, 115, 116, 117
bronchial carcinoma, 112

C

cancer stem cell(s), xiii 84, 88, 113
carcinogenesis, 18, 1110
cell cycle, 5, 6, 8, 9, 27, 29, 42, 49, 53, 56, 63, 75, 80, 81, 90, 94, 101, 106, 110, 111, 112, 118

cell death, 5, 6, 7, 9, 11, 27, 30, 42, 44, 50, 51, 53, 63, 66, 76, 77, 84, 94, 100, 102, 109, 114, 115
cell line(s), 6, 42, 46, 49, 50, 51, 56, 62, 63, 64, 65, 75, 77, 80, 81, 84, 91, 94, 112, 116, 117
cervical cancer, 2, 28, 30, 31, 48, 49, 53, 57, 58, 60, 66, 67, 71, 113, 116
chemotherapy, ix, 1, 2, 47, 50, 52, 82, 121
childhood ependymoma, 12
Chinese medicine, 80, 85
Chinese traditional medicine, 91
chronic myelogenous leukemia, 29, 30, 53, 59, 62
clinical outcome, viii, xi, 10, 65, 105, 108
clinical trials, 43, 53, 65, 67, 84, 92, 95, 107
clonogenic assay, 6, 27
cocoa, 22, 63
coffee, 24, 79
colon cancer, 28, 55, 68, 73, 75, 79, 10o, 102, 116
colorectal cancer, 2, 31, 50, 51, 54, 60, 61, 62, 67, 68, 71, 75, 81, 110, 115, 116, 117
complementary treatments, vii, x
cyclooxygenase, xiii, 49
cytotoxicity, 74, 80, 110

D

diet, 20, 55, 60, 79
dietary habits, 50
dietary supplements, 20, 52, 56, 108, 110
DNA damage, 6, 8, 9, 13, 28, 29, 30, 33, 39, 46, 48, 51, 54, 56, 63, 65, 72, 73, 79, 80, 83, 86, 87, 90, 94, 95, 102
DNA double strand breaks (DSBs), 6, 8, 9, 37, 39, 42, 46, 66, 90, 99, 100, 116
DNA repair, 5, 6, 8, 9, 14, 18, 30, 33, 35, 42, 46, 48, 51, 65, 66, 67, 75, 98, 106, 111, 114
DNA strand breaks, 5, 74

dosage, vii, 107, 108
doxorubicin, 100, 102, 115

E

Ehrlich carcinoma, 83, 86, 110
endothelial cells, 14, 62, 113
eosinophilic leukemia, 59, 62
ependymoma, 12
epithelial-mesenchymal transition (EMT), xiv, 8, 14, 15, 72, 73, 77, 78, 86, 87, 88, 91, 92, 93, 95, 112, 114
esophageal cancer, 2, 28, 31, 50, 53, 55, 56, 88, 91, 112, 116
estrogen, xiv, 47, 53, 66, 117

F

fibroblast(s), 45, 63, 65, 78, 94
fibrosis, 2, 40, 42, 47
food, x, 17, 20, 121, 122
fractionated irradiation, 37, 43, 69, 72
free radical(s), 5, 6, 18, 56, 108
fruits, 19, 23, 24, 25, 63, 64, 67, 75, 76, 79, 81, 83, 90, 91, 107

G

gastric cancer, 2, 84, 85, 88, 91, 93, 110, 113
genomic instability, 9
genotoxic stress, 8, 9, 10, 42
glioblastoma, 2, 3, 11, 30, 52, 54, 59, 61, 62, 63, 64, 65, 70, 108, 114, 117, 118
glioblastoma multiforme, 30, 52
glioma, 12, 62, 64
green tea, 20, 22, 56, 57, 58, 61, 62, 63, 64, 106, 113, 114, 117, 119

H

head and neck tumors, 82
hematopoietic stem cells, 53
hepatocellular carcinoma, 51, 67, 83, 100, 105, 112
hepatoma, 32, 51, 67, 71, 83, 87, 99, 103, 114,
herb(s), x, 17, 23, 25, 55, 76, 83, 90
homeostasis, 10
homologous recombination (HRR), xiv, 9, 33, 35, 42, 51
hormonal treatment, 47
HPV16, 31, 48
HPV18, 49, 66
HPV39, 28, 31, 48
human papillomavirus (HPV), xiv, 28, 30, 48, 49, 58, 66
hyper-radiosensitivity (HRS), xiv, 34, 35, 43
hypertension, 44
hypoxia, xiv, 14, 18, 82, 114

I

in vitro, 6, 40, 41, 42, 43, 49, 53, 62, 67, 85, 93, 97, 100, 107, 109, 110, 112, 113, 114, 116, 115, 118, 119,
in vivo, 6, 40, 42, 49, 53, 58, 65, 67, 76, 77, 82, 83, 85, 92, 93, 95, 96, 99, 101, 105, 107, 108, 110, 111, 115, 116, 117
incidence, vii, ix, 1, 20, 43, 44, 45, 47, 48, 50, 51, 55, 63, 84, 93, 109
inflammatory cells, 40, 42
ingestion, 21, 107
invasion, 15, 57, 88, 95, 97, 98
ionizing radiation, vii, x, 1, 3, 5, 6, 7, 8, 9, 10, 12, 13, 14, 15, 18, 19, 20, 41, 43, 45, 46, 51, 52, 54, 57, 58, 62, 63, 65, 66, 80, 84, 85, 90, 92, 95, 96, 99, 101, 104, 106, 108, 113, 114, 117

irradiation, viii, x, xi, 2, 3, 6, 9, 15, 27, 28, 29, 30, 31, 32, 33, 34, 35, 36, 37, 38, 39, 40, 41, 42, 43, 48, 49, 51, 52, 53, 59, 60, 61, 62, 63, 64, 65, 68, 69, 70, 71, 72, 73, 74, 76, 83, 86, 87, 88, 90, 91, 93, 95, 97, 98, 99, 101, 102, 103, 105, 106, 116,

K

kidney cancer, 32, 44

L

laryngeal cancer, 82, 86, 115
leukemia(s), xiv, 2, 29, 30, 53, 54, 59, 62, 108
lifestyle, ix, 1, 50
liver cancer, 32, 99, 102, 104
lung cancer, 1, 2, 10, 32, 33, 39, 45, 46, 53, 69, 72, 73, 76, 77, 78, 82, 84, 85, 86, 87, 89, 90, 91, 92, 93, 96, 97, 109, 111, 112, 114, 116, 117
lymphoma(s), xiii, 2

M

matrix metalloproteinase (MMP), xv, 8, 15, 57, 60, 83, 86, 89, 93, 95, 97, 98
medulloblastoma, 65, 70, 113
metabolic conversion, 107
metabolites, x, 20, 121
metastasis, 3, 13, 15, 17, 29, 36, 38, 39, 40, 41, 42, 43, 44, 57, 89, 93
metastatic spread, 40, 41, 42, 44, 93, 106
microenvironment, 3, 42, 82
microRNA (miR), xiv, 72, 73, 77, 86, 87, 88, 91, 92, 112
migration, 15, 44, 77, 87, 95, 97, 98

model(s), vii, 20, 40, 41, 43, 44, 46, 49, 52, 55, 57, 58, 66, 67, 77, 92, 99, 105, 107, 111, 112, 113, 117
mortality, 17, 45, 63, 95, 109
multiple myeloma, 59, 62
myeloid leukemia, 29, 54, 108

N

necrosis, xv, 40
necrotic death, 62
neutron irradiation, 27, 34
non-homologous end joining (NHEJ), xv, 9, 33, 35, 37, 42
non-small cell lung cancer, 2, 10, 32, 33, 39, 45, 46, 53, 69, 72, 73, 76, 77, 78, 82, 84, 85, 86, 87, 89, 90, 91, 93, 96, 109, 111, 112, 114, 117
Notch, 15, 72, 73, 77, 78, 86, 87, 88, 91, 92, 93, 106, 112
Nrf2, xv, 7, 8, 28, 33, 45, 56, 60, 61, 99, 102, 106, 115
nuclear factor-κB (NF-κB), xv, 8, 12, 13, 14, 18, 27, 29, 33, 34, 35, 36, 37, 38, 39, 41, 42, 46, 57, 60, 68, 72, 73, 77, 81, 86, 87, 92, 96, 97, 114
nutritional supplements, x

O

obesity, 44
oral cancer, 2, 60, 61, 63, 84, 85, 88, 109, 113
ovarian cancer, 66, 67, 72, 109
overall survival, 2, 11, 96
oxidative damage, 18, 33, 45, 99, 102
oxidative stress, 7, 28, 45, 56, 73, 79, 94, 95, 97, 99, 102

P

p53, 8, 11, 31, 32, 45, 48, 49, 50, 66, 72, 73, 75, 77, 78, 84, 86, 87, 91, 100, 109, 112, 113
pancreatic cancer, 2, 3, 10, 59, 63
phosphorylation, 7, 8, 12, 31, 59, 60, 63, 68, 69, 87, 116
photon irradiation, 27, 28, 29, 30, 31, 32, 33, 34, 35, 36, 37, 38, 44, 59, 69
physical activity, 50
phytochemical(s), vii, x, 17, 18, 19, 67, 110
PI3K, xv, 8, 12, 13, 18, 69, 76, 82, 96, 115
plant polyphenols, vii, x, 18, 117
pneumonitis, 2, 47
polyphenol(s), vii, x, 18, 20, 56, 57, 62, 114, 118, 121
primary tumor, 40, 41, 43, 44
progesterone, 47
prognosis, 11, 48, 51, 52, 57, 61
proliferation, 6, 13, 28, 31, 34, 40, 43, 47, 52, 55, 57, 59, 60, 61, 62, 68, 69, 72, 73, 75, 76, 77, 86, 87, 91, 102, 104, 106, 114
prooxidant(s), 18, 55, 99, 106
prostaglandin, xv, 49, 85
prostate cancer, 1, 2, 9, 10, 14, 20, 26, 27, 29, 33, 34, 35, 36, 37, 38, 40, 41, 42, 43, 44, 53, 58, 60, 63, 74, 80, 94, 95, 96, 97, 98, 108, 111, 114, 115, 117, 118
protein kinase B (Akt), xiii, xv, 8, 12, 13, 18, 31, 50, 51, 57, 60, 65, 69, 70, 75, 76, 80, 82, 85, 87, 90, 93, 95, 96, 97, 101, 106, 108, 111, 115, 117, 118
public health, vii, 26

Q

quality of life, xi, 2, 75, 106, 108

Index

R

radiation, vii, ix, x, 1, 2, 3, 5, 6, 7, 8, 9, 10, 11, 12, 13, 14, 15, 17, 19, 20, 27, 29, 30, 31, 33, 34, 35, 37, 38, 39, 40, 41, 42, 43, 44, 45, 46, 47, 48, 49, 50, 51, 52, 53, 54, 55, 56, 57, 58, 59, 60, 61, 62, 63, 64, 65, 66, 67, 68, 69, 70, 71, 72, 73, 74, 75, 76, 77, 78, 79, 80, 81, 82, 83, 84, 85, 86, 87, 88, 89, 90, 91, 92, 93, 94, 95, 96, 97, 98, 99, 100, 101, 102, 104, 106, 107, 108, 110, 111, 112, 113, 114, 115, 116, 117, 118, 119
radiation therapy, 1, 7, 9, 10, 18, 53, 111
radioprotector, 52, 58, 63
radioresistance, v, ix, x, xi, 3, 5, 6, 7, 8, 10, 11, 12, 13, 14, 18, 43, 53, 58, 77, 82, 83, 84, 91, 95, 96, 106
radiosensitivity, x, xiv, 9, 11, 13, 14, 28, 45, 46, 48, 49, 50, 53, 55, 59, 65, 67, 71, 75, 76, 78, 82, 83, 92, 97, 99, 101, 109, 110, 111, 112, 113, 114, 115, 116, 118
radiosensitization, 7, 9, 13, 18, 46, 84, 86, 100, 106, 107, 109, 110, 112, 114, 115, 117
radiosensitizer(s), vii, x, xi, 3, 4, 6, 8, 11, 12, 17, 18, 42, 43, 48, 52, 56, 64, 65, 67, 75, 76, 78, 82, 83, 84, 85, 90, 91, 92, 95, 99, 100, 108, 109, 112, 113, 117
radiotherapy, v, vii, viii, ix, x, xi, 1, 2, 3, 5, 8, 9, 10, 11, 12, 14, 15, 17, 19, 26, 43, 44, 47, 48, 50, 51, 52, 54, 57, 58, 60, 61, 63, 64, 79, 80, 82, 84, 90, 100, 105, 106, 108, 110, 111, 112, 113, 116, 117, 121
radiotoxicity, 55, 58, 61, 63, 67, 80, 109, 114
reactive oxygen species (ROS), xv, 5, 6, 7, 18, 28, 31, 33, 45, 49, 55, 56, 58, 74, 80, 84, 87, 94, 98, 99, 102, 109
recurrence, 2, 3, 6, 11, 13
red wine, 23, 78
redox imbalance, 99
redox status, vii, 7, 8, 45, 99, 106, 110, 115
relapse, 2, 3, 15
renal cell carcinoma, 32, 44, 53, 118
risk factors, 1, 44

S

safety, x, 18, 106, 107
sarcoma, xiv, 37, 51, 52, 116
side effects, 3, 5
smoking, 44
soft tissue sarcoma, 51, 52
solid tumor(s), 2, 67, 83, 85
soy, 20, 21, 37, 38, 40, 41, 42, 43, 46, 49, 53, 54, 105, 106, 110, 111, 112, 117,
soybeans, 20, 21, 22
squamous cell carcinoma, 2, 50, 53, 56, 60, 61, 82, 84, 85, 88, 91, 112
surgery, 1, 2, 47, 50, 52
surgical resection, ix, 2, 48, 82
survival rate, 2, 43, 82
survival time, xi, 109

T

taxanes, 3
therapeutic outcome, x, 2, 3, 4, 6, 12, 43, 50, 53, 64, 67, 78

V

vascular endothelial growth factor (VEGF), xv, 14, 38, 57, 60, 83, 85, 86, 87, 95, 97
vegetables, 19, 23, 24, 25, 63, 64, 67, 75, 76, 79, 81, 84

X

xenograft(s), 12, 40, 43, 44, 46, 56, 66, 67, 68, 75, 76, 77, 81, 82, 84, 92, 93, 95, 96, 99, 113

x-ray, 5, 29, 30, 31, 32, 33, 34, 35, 37, 39, 59, 60, 68, 69, 71, 72, 73, 86, 87, 88, 89, 102, 103, 114, 118

Γ

γ-H2AX, 8, 46, 66, 67, 68, 71, 72, 90, 94, 98

Related Nova Publications

THE STORY OF HYDRA: PORTRAIT OF CANCER AS A STEM-CELL DISEASE

AUTHOR: Shi-Ming Tu, MD

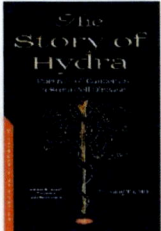

SERIES: Cancer Etiology, Diagnosis and Treatments

BOOK DESCRIPTION: The questions we ask in this book about cancer are actually quite elementary. What is the origin of cancer? Does cancer arise in any cell in the body, or only in certain cells? Is cancer a genetic or a stem-cell disease?

HARDCOVER ISBN: 978-1-53615-373-6
RETAIL PRICE: $230

CLINICAL ONCOPROTEOMICS: PROTEOME-BASED PERSONALIZED ANTI-CANCER THERAPY

AUTHOR: Andrey S. Bryukhovetskiy, M.D., Ph.D.

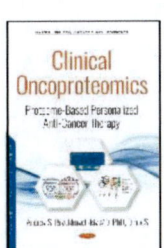

SERIES: Cancer Etiology, Diagnosis and Treatments

BOOK DESCRIPTION: This book reviews various academic viewpoints on the informational component and value of the data of clinical oncoproteomics for the diagnostics and treatment of malignant tumors using cellular, genomic and post-genomic technologies.

HARDCOVER ISBN: 978-1-53614-477-2
RETAIL PRICE: $230

To see a complete list of Nova publications, please visit our website at www.novapublishers.com

Related Nova Publications

PENILE CANCER: CHALLENGES AND CONTROVERSIES

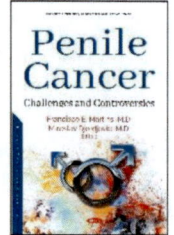

EDITORS: Francisco E. Martins, MD and Miroslav L. Djordjevic, MD, PhD

SERIES: Cancer Etiology, Diagnosis and Treatments

BOOK DESCRIPTION: This book, with its multidisciplinary approach, is intended to provide a comprehensive discussion and benefit every reader, junior or senior, world over who is interested in and deals with patients afflicted by penile cancer, including the urologic oncologist, the radiation oncologist, the medical oncologist, the urology resident, and last but not least the primary care physician.

HARDCOVER ISBN: 978-1-53615-950-9
RETAIL PRICE: $230

ENCYCLOPEDIA OF BREAST CANCER: NEW RESEARCH (3 VOLUME SET)

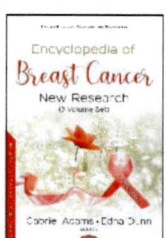

EDITORS: Gabriel Adams and Edna Dunn

SERIES: Cancer Etiology, Diagnosis and Treatments

BOOK DESCRIPTION: This 3 volume set covers a wide range of topics, including:
· gemcitabine
· oophorectomies
· breast cancer growth inhibition
· exosomes
· tumor infiltrating lymphocytes

HARDCOVER ISBN: 978-1-53615-697-3
RETAIL PRICE: $495

To see a complete list of Nova publications, please visit our website at www.novapublishers.com